Respiratory Care

an Oakes Pocket Guide

9th Edition

Dana F. Oakes
Scot N. Jones

RespiratoryBooks

a division of:
Health Educator Publications, Inc.
476 Shotwell Road
Suite 102, PMB 161
Clayton, NC 27520

DANA F. OAKES BA, RRT-NPS
Educational Consultant

Formerly:
Director of Clinical Education
Respiratory Care Program
Columbia Union College
Tacoma Park, Maryland

Educational Coordinator/Instructor
Respiratory Care Department
Children's Hospital Nat. Medical Center
Washington, D.C.

Director of Respiratory Care
VA Medical Center
Washington, D.C.

SCOT JONES BA, RRT-ACCS
Educational Consultant

Formerly:
Director of Clinical Education
Respiratory Care Program
Broward College
Coconut Creek, Florida

Respiratory Care Supervisor
Respiratory Care Department
Vidant Medical Center
Greenville, NC

Copyright © 2017
9th edition
Health Educator Publications, Inc.
Copyright under the Uniform Copyright Convention. All rights reserved. No part of this book may be reproduced, stored in a retrieval system, or transmitted in any form or by any means, electronic, mechanical, photocopying, recording or otherwise, without written permission of the Publisher.
Printed in China

ISBN 978-0-932887-58-0

RespiratoryBooks
A Division of Health Educator Publications, Inc.
476 Shotwell Drive, PMB 161
Clayton, NC 27520

The Authors and Publisher has exerted every effort to ensure that the clinical principles, procedures, and practices described herein are based on current knowledge and state-of-the-art information available from acknowledged authorities, texts, and journals. Nevertheless, they cannot be considered absolute and universal recommendations. Each patient situation must be considered individually. The Authors and Publisher disclaim responsibility for any adverse effects resulting directly or indirectly from information presented in this book, undetected errors, or misunderstandings by the readers.

Table of Contents
(detailed table of contents at start of each chapter).

Important Disclaimer:

The Author and Publisher has exerted every effort to ensure that the clinical principles, procedures, and practices described herein are based on current knowledge and state-of-the-art information available from acknowledged authorities, texts, and journals. Nevertheless, they cannot be considered absolute and universal recommendations. Each patient situation must be considered individually. The reader is urged to check the package inserts of drugs and disposable equipment and the manufacturer's manual of durable equipment for indications, contraindications, proper usage, warnings, and precautions before use. The Author and Publisher disclaim responsibility for any adverse effects resulting directly or indirectly from information presented in this book, undetected errors, or misunderstandings by the readers.

Acknowledgement

Always first and foremost, we are thankful for our Lord, Jesus Christ, for His allowing us to play this small part in our field, for guiding our hands for over 30 years, for the tens of thousands that have used this pocket guide clinically. To Him, and to Him only goes the Glory.

An Open Invitation

We know that the books are what they are today in part due to the feedback of clinicians, clinician educators, and students. Please consider this an open invitation to provide us with your thoughts on what you like, what you would like to see improved, or anything in between!

Email: Scot Jones scot.jones@respiratorybooks.com
        Dana Oakes danaoakes@respiratorybooks.com

1 | Patient Assessment

Selected Health History	
Obtain and/or Review the following (not just respiratory):	
Demographics	Name, gender, age, occupation
Chief Complaint	The primary reason(s) the person has presented for care
History of Present Illness (HPI)	Chronological description of: Each Symptom (see pg 1-15); Onset; Location (Radiating?); Timing (Freq, Duration); Character (Quality, Quantity, Severity)
Past Medical History	Including childhood diseases, all significant illnesses/injuries, and hospitalizations. Include those untreated
Family	Four generations of all illnesses/diseases
Social	Hobbies, recreation, living arrangements, social activities, habits, substance abuse, and travel

(Continued Next Page)

Emotional	Satisfaction with life, stress, relationships, finances, psychiatric illnesses
Occupational Environmental	**Work or Live Around:** Farms, Foundries, Mills, Mines, Shipyards, Asbestos, Dust, Fumes, Gases, Smoke, Toxic Chemicals, etc. **Home Irritants:** Air conditioning, Glue, Humidifiers, Insulation, Paint, Pets, Smoking, Woodpiles, Mold **Geographic fungi (region)** See Ch 11: Histoplasmosis, Asbestosis, Aspergillis, etc.
Cardio-pulmonary **Pack Years =** (# Yrs Smoked) X (# Packs/Day)	**Pulmonary:** Allergies, Asthma, Bronchiectasis, CA, Colds, COPD, CF, Fungal Infections, Influenza, Lupus, PNA, Pneumothorax, Pleurisy, Sinus Infections, Sleep Apneas, Alpha-1, etc. **Cardiovascular:** CHD, Diabetes, MI, Heart Failure, HTN, Obesity, Surgery, Trauma **Drug Abuse:** There is often a correlation between respiratory problems and illicit drug abuse. Encourage honesty **Habits:** Alcohol, Diet, Exercise, Sleep
Review of Systems	A list of questions looking at body systems to uncover problems related to Chief Complaint (CC)
Cardio Care/ Medications	All current drugs (include OTC, natural) Any current pulmonary treatments
Review of Physician's Orders and/or Relevant Protocols	

Respectful Bedside Assessment

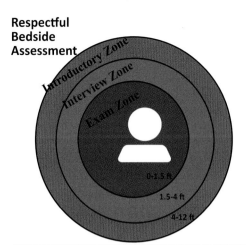

Introductory Zone
Interview Zone
Exam Zone

0-1.5 ft
1.5-4 ft
4-12 ft

Introduction (establish a positive rapport, obtain patient's cooperation, determine overall patient condition, assess environment for safety)
- Address pt. by formal name - avoid extremes in friendliness
- Introduce Yourself; Explain your professional role and state purpose of visit
- Be warm, friendly, and professional (clean, neat, eye contact)

Interview (obtain information concerning CC and further develop positive rapport)
- Provide necessary privacy
- Use appropriate eye contact, and avoid standing at foot of bed
- Maintain a relaxed style; be honest; communicate empathy
- Never argue or make moral judgments
- Use Interpreter if needed, use non-medical language (no jargon)

Physical Exam (determine condition of patient and insure prescribed treatment is appropriate)
- Request permission to check ID and to perform exam
- Use minimal/no eye contact, only necessary touch, min. verbal
- Be aware of patient's response
- Use appropriate PPE to establish professional/infectious barriers

ASSESSMENT

Inspection

General Appearance

- Age
- Weight
- Height
- Body Structure
- Skin Color
- Hygiene
- Culture
- Level of Distress
- Motor Activity
- Nutrition
- Physical limitations
- Sensory limitations

Mental Status

Level of Consciousness
(see details on pg 1-21)

- Anxiety
- Restlessness
- Altered Speech
- Confusion
- Disorientation

Cardiopulmonary Distress

Anxiety
- Cool Hands
- Sweaty Palms
- Fidgety
- Restless
- Tense

Body Position
- Leaning on elbows?

Chest Pain
- Guarding
- Moaning
- Shallow Breaths
- Writhing

Breathing
- Choking
- Gurgling
- Coughing
- Dyspnea
- Irregular Pattern
- Labored
- Rapid
- Shallow
- Wheezing

see pg 1-11 for breathing patterns

Personality and Attitude

- Responses towards their illness
- Responses towards you
- Resistive
- Crossed Arms
- Lack of Eye Contact
- Brief, Curt Responses

Vital Signs: Normal and Abnormal Ranges

See Oakes' Hemodynamic Monitoring for detailed instructions on Pulse and BP monitoring

Age	Respiratory Rate	Heart Rate	Blood Pressure
Adult	12-16	60-100	110-120/70-80
5-12 yrs	16-20	70-110	100/60
1-4 yrs	20-30	80-120	95/50
1st year	25-40	80-160	85/50
Newborn	30-60	90-180	75/40
Adult Abnormal ranges	< 12 = bradypnea > 20 = tachypnea	< 60 = bradycardia > 100 = tachycardia	< 90/60 = hypotension > 140/90 = hypertension
Notes	See page 1-11 for respiratory patterns	Pulse deficit = difference between auscultated beats and peripheral pulse Check equality of pulse strengths in all major arteries: Right vs. Left Upper vs. Lower extremities Inspiration vs. Expiration	Mean BP = BPsys + 2 BPdia / 3 (adult normal = 93) Pulse Pressure (PP) = BPsys - BPdia (adult normal = 40)

Strength (amplitude) of Pulse

4 - bounding	1 - diminished
3 - full, increased	0 - absent
2 - normal	

Heart Rhythms

Pulsus Alternans	Regular alteration of weak and strong pulses
Pulsus Corrigans	Strong or Bounding, with ↑PP
Pulsus Parvus	Weak Pulse with ↓PP
Pulsus Paradoxus	↓ Pulse Strength during Inspiration; ↑ during Expiration (> 10 mmHg is signif., > 20 is needed to feel the difference)
Reverse Pulsus Paradoxus	Reverse of above - as noted during Positive Pressure Ventilation

Pulse Oximetry (SpO$_2$)

	Normal	Hypoxemia		
		Mild	Moderate	Severe
Adult	95-99%	91-94%	76-90%	< 75%
Child	91-96%	88-90%	76-87%	< 75%

Pulse Oximetry Quick Troubleshooting	
Check:	• Good Perfusion? • Good Waveform? • Skin Temperature at Probe? • Ambient Light or Nailpolish?
Try:	• Switch position or type of probe • Replace probe • Cover probe (if bright room) • Warm body part with approved heat pack • Verify using ABG if necessary

Temperature

Core (Most Accurate)	Intermediate (Affected by Body, Environment)
• Pulmonary Artery • Esophageal Probe • Nasopharynx • Tympanic (Ear) • Jugular Bulb	• Sublingual (under tongue) • Axillary (under arm) • Rectal • Forehead • Bladder

Normal Temperature Ranges

Place	Celsius Range	Fahrenheit Range
Core	36.5 – 37.5° C	97.7 – 99.5° F
Oral*	36.5 – 37.5° C	97.7 – 99.5° F
Axillary	35.9 – 36.9° C	96.7 – 98.5° F
Otic (tympanic)	37.1 – 38.1° C	98.7 – 100.5° F

*Cool or heated aerosol may affect temperature readings

Select Causes of Abnormal Temperatures
(defined as those outside of the above Normal Temp Ranges)

Hypothermia	Hyperthermia (rapid onset, diffic. to control, doesn't respond to antipyretics)
• Environmental Exposure • Extremes of Age • Brain/Spinal Injuries • Shock • Anesthesia • Sedation • Therapeutic (MI)	• Environmental Exposure • Malignant (Drug-Related) • Brain/Spinal Injuries
	Fever (usually responds to antipyretics)
	• Infection (w/ ↑ WBC)

Thoracic Cage Landmarks

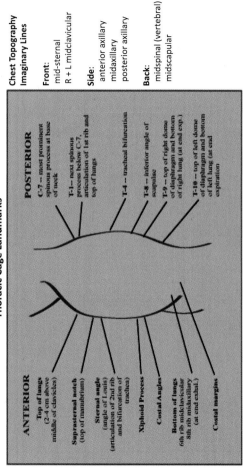

ANTERIOR

Top of lungs (2-4 cm above middle of clavicles)

Suprasternal notch (top of manubrium)

Sternal angle (angle of Louis) (articulation of 2nd rib and bifurcation of trachea)

Xiphoid Process

Costal Angles

Bottom of lungs 6th rib midclavicular 8th rib midaxillary (at end exhal.)

Costal margins

POSTERIOR

C-7 – most prominent spinous process at base of neck

T-1 – next spinous process below C-7, articulation of 1st rib and top of lungs

T-4 – tracheal bifurcation

T-8 – inferior angle of scapulae

T-9 – top of right dome of diaphragm and bottom of right lung (at end exp.)

T-10 – top of left dome of diaphragm and bottom of left lung (at end expiration)

Chest Topography Imaginary Lines

Front:
mid-sternal
R + L midclavicular

Side:
anterior axillary
midaxillary
posterior axillary

Back:
midspinal (vertebral)
midscapular

1-8

Topographic Position of the Lungs and Heart

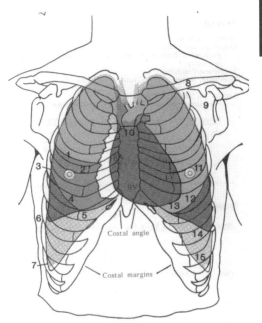

1. Transverse fissure
2. 4th rib midclavicular
3. Oblique fissure at
   5th rib midaxillary
4. Oblique fissure
5. Lung border during expir-
   ation(6th rib midclav)
6. Lung border during expir-
   ation(8th rib mid axill)
7. Pleural border (10th rib
   midaxillary)
8. Clavicle

9. Scapula
10. Aorta
11. Nipple (4th intercostal
    space in male)
12. Oblique fissure
13. Apex of heart (PMI at
    5th intercostal space)
14. Lung border during expir-
    ation(8th rib midaxillary)
15. Pleural border (10th rib
    midaxillary)

Head and Neck

Head	Neck
Face: Color, facial expression (alert, distress, fear, mood, pain) **Nose**: Nasal flaring **Lips**: Color, pursed lip breathing **Eyes**: Pupillary reflexes Mydriasis = fixed & dilate Miosis = pinpoint	**Accessory muscle use** (↑sternocleidomastoid =↑WOB) **Carotid pulse** **Jugular vein distention** (JVD) **Lymphadenopathy** (infection, HIV) **Tracheal position** see pg 1-12

Chest Shape

Diameter	Rib Angles	Symmetry
Normal AP diameter = 1/2 to 2/3 (> 2/3 = barrel chest)	Normal = 45° COPD = horizontal	Flail chest Pneumothorax Splinting

Deformities:
Lesions, obesity, muscular atrophy/hypertrophy, rib fractures, scars, spine (kyphosis, scoliosis), sternum (pectus carinatum/excavatum)

Breathing Rate (see Pg. 1-5)
Breathing Pattern (see also next page)

I/E Ratio
 Posture
 SOB (dyspnea while talking,
   nasal flaring, pursed-lip)
 Orthopnea = SOB lying down
 Platypnea = SOB upright
 Accessory muscle use:
   substernal, suprasternal, in
   tercostal, bulging, retrac
   tions, clavicular lift, splinting
 Symmetry – uni or bilateral
	Abdominal distension
	   (ascites, obesity, pregnancy)
	 Excursion (depth):
	   Chest vs. abdomen
	 Respiratory alternans–
	   chest wall breathing
	   alternating with dia
	   phragm breathing
	 Paradoxical (flail chest)
	 Abdominal paradox
	   (abdomen inward during
	   inspiration)

Restriction: Typically rapid/shallow breathing
Obstruction: Typically ↑T_E = lower airway; ↑T_I = upper airway
Paroxysmal Nocturnal Dyspnea (PND) = SOB and coughing
(generally at night)

Breathing Patterns

Type	Pattern	Characteristics	Causes
Eupnea		Normal rate (12 - 20 bpm) Normal rhythm, Sighs 7/hr	Normal physiology
Apnea		Absence of breathing	Respiratory or cardiac arrest, ↑ICP
Bradypnea		Slow rate (< 10 bpm), regular rhythm	Normal during sleep, brain tumors, diabetic coma, drugs (alcohol, narcotics), ↑ICP, metabolic alkalosis (limited), uremia
Tachypnea		↑ Rate (> 25 bpm), regular rhythm	Anxiety (esp. asthmatics), atelectasis, brain lesions, drugs (aspirin), exercise, fear, fever, hypercapnia, hypoxemia, hypoxia, metabolic acidosis, obesity, pain
Hypopnea		↓ Depth, normal rate, regular rhythm	Circulatory failure, meningitis, unconsciousness
Hyperpnea		↑ Depth, normal rate, regular rhythm	Exertion, fever, pain, respiratory disease
Apneustic		Long gasping inspirations with insufficient expiration	Lesions in the pneumotaxic center
Biot's		Fast and deep breaths with periods of apnea, no set rhythm	Spinal meningitis, ↑ICP, CNS lesions or disease
Cheynes-Stokes		↑ Breaths (rate & depth) then decreasing breaths followed by periods of apnea (20-60 sec)	Normal in newborns and aged, CHF, aortic valve lesion, dissecting aneurysm, ↑CO2 sensitivity meningitis, ↑ICP, cerebral anoxia, drug overdose (morphine), renal failure
Kussmaul's		Fast and deep breaths like sighs with no expiratory phase	DKA, severe hemorrhage, peritonitis, renal failure, uremia

Palpation

Tracheal Position (shift from midline)	Chest & Diaphragm Excursion
Shift towards: unlateral upper lobe collapse **Shift away**: lung tumor, pleural effusion, tension pneumothorax	**Normal**: 3 cm women, 4-6 cm men (posteriorly) **Unilateral** ↓: atelectasis, lobar consolidation, pleural effusion, pneumothorax **Bilateral** ↓: COPD, NM disease

Tactile (vocal) fremitus	Skin
feeling vocal vibrations when patient says "99" with a low-pitched voice	bruises, masses, subcutaneous emphysema, turgor
	PMI, Tenderness, fractures

↓ Fremitus Vibrations	↑ Fremitus Vibrations
Airflow↓: Obstruction (COPD, secretions), restriction (shallow breathing), ET tube malposition **Barrier**: Air – COPD, pneumothorax Fat – Obesity Fibrosis – Pleural thickening Fluid – Pleural effusion Muscle – Hypertrophy	**Consolidation:** Atelectasis Fibrosis Infarct Pneumonia Tumor

Percussion

Note	Normal Areas	Abnormal Areas
Flat	Thigh, muscle	Massive atelectasis or pleural effusion, pneumonectomy
Dull	Heart, liver	Atelectasis, consolid., enlarged heart, fibrosis, neoplasm, pleural effusion or thicken., pulm. edema
Resonance	Normal lung	
Hyper-resonance	Abdomen	Acute asthma, emphysema, pneumothorax
Tympany	Large gastric air bubble	Large pulmonary cavity, tension pneumothorax

Auscultation

Normal Breath Sounds

Type	Description	I:E
Vesicular	Normal sound over most of lungs	3:1 breezy
Bronchovesicular	Normal sound over carina area and between upper scapulae	1:1 breezy/ tubular
Bronchial	Normal sound over manubrium	2:3 hollow/tubular/loud
Tracheal	Normal sound over upper trachea	5:6 tubular/loud/harsh

Abnormal Breath Sounds (see also Adventitious, next page)

↓ Breath Sounds	↑Breath Sounds
Airflow ↓: Obstruction (COPD, secretions), restriction (shallow breathing), ET tube malpositioned **Barrier:** Air – COPD, pneumothorax Fat – Obesity Fibrosis – Pleural thickening; Fluid – Pleural effusion Muscle – Hypertrophy	**Consolidation:** Atelectasis Fibrosis Infarct Pneumonia Tumor

Voice Sounds (Vocal Resonance)

Type	Normal	Abnormal
Bronchophony	Spoken syllables are non-distinct	↑ distinction = consolidation
Whispered pectoriloquy	Whispers are faint & non-distinct	↓ distinction = air or fluid insulation
Egophony	Spoken E → E	Spoken E→ A = lung consolid over a pleural effusion

Adventitious Breath Sounds *

Type	Description	Probable Location	Common Causes
Crackle – Discontinuous vibrations	*Fine* – High-pitched crackling at end inspiration *Medium* – Wetter and louder at any part of inspiration *Coarse* – Loud, low-pitched bubbling at expiration or inspir.	*Alveoli* – Atelectasis or excessive fluid *Bronchioles* – Air moving through fluid *Larger airways* – Air moving through fluid, may clear w/ cough	Atelectasis, fibrosis, pneumonia, pulmonary edema Bronchitis, emphysema, pneumonia, pulmonary edema Bronchitis, emphysema, pneumonia, pulmonary edema
Wheeze – Continuous vibrations	Musical – usually occurs during expiration, but may occur during inspiration	*High pitch:* Lower airway squeak due to narrowing *Low pitch* (rhonchi): Upper airway snore (usually due to sputum production that may disappear with cough)	Asthma, bronchitis, CHF, emphysema, foreign body, mucous plug, stenosis, tumor
Stridor – Continuous vibrations	Loud, high-pitched crowing in upper airway, usually during inspiration	Usually due to upper airway obstruction (usually inspir = above glottis; expir = lower trachea)	Croup, epiglottitis, foreign body, tracheal stenosis, tumor, vocal cord edema
Rub – Pleural or pericardial	Grating vibration, loud & harsh *Pleural:* Assoc. with I & E *Pericardial:* Assoc. with heart beat	*Pleural* – pleural membrane rub *Pericardial* – pericardial sac rub	Pleurisy, peripheral pneumonia, pulmonary emboli, TB Pericarditis

* As recommended by ACCP-ATS Joint Committee on Pulmonary Nomenclature, 1975 and updates

Other Respiratory Assessments

Fingers	Tremors, Yellow Stains, Clubbing (see Ch 11)
Sputum	See Ch 5
Skin and Mucous Membranes	
Capillary Refill	Pinch fingernail for 5 sec: Normal = color returns to fingernail ≤ 3 sec > 3 sec = ↓CO or poor digital perfusion.
Temperature	Cold (cool room, ↓ circulation) Warm/flushed (warm room, anxiety, embarrassment, fever, hypercapnia)
Rashes, bruises, lesions	Note age of bruising, lesions. Ask about Rashes - New? Medication related?
Color	Pallor, Flush, Cyanosis
Peripheral	(acrocyanosis) - Poor Circulation
Central Cyanosis	Poor Blood Oxygen.
Edema	Legs, Ankles ⟶

Pitting Scale	
1+	rapid
2+	10-15 seconds
3+	1-2 minutes
4+	> 2 minutes

Pulmonary Symptoms: Questions to Consider

1. **Cough:** Note sound, productive, frequency, duration, onset, triggers, severity

2. **Dyspnea:** Note inspiratory (↑ airway) vs expiratory (↓ airway), Orthopnea, Platypnea, frequency and duration, onset, triggers, severity

3. **Chest Pain:** Note if pleuritic, frequency and duration, location and radiation, triggers, severity

4. **Hemoptysis:** Note amount, odor, frequency and duration, severity (massive = 300 mL in 3 hrs or 600 mL in 24 hrs). See Chapter 5

Common Disease Assessment Findings

Disease		Palpation		Auscultation
Asthma	↑RR, ↑TE, dyspnea, ↑accessory muscle use, nasal flaring, orthopnea, ↑A-P diameter	Normal or ↓ fremitus	Normal or hyper resonance (?)	↓BS (severe ↓ = danger), wheezes, crackles, ↑TE
Atelectasis	↑RR, dyspnea, ↓ chest expansion (same side), tracheal deviation (same side)	↑ fremitus	Dull	↑ or ↓BS, crackles (fine), whispered pectoriloquy
Chronic Bronchitis	↑RR, ↑TE, dyspnea, ↑accessory muscle use, fat or stocky, ↑A-P diameter, chronic cough, cyanosis, ↓ diaphragm movement	Normal or ↓ fremitus	Normal to dull	↓BS, crackles (all types), wheeze
Emphysema	↑RR, ↑TE, dyspnea, orthopnea, pursed-lip breathing, hypertrophy of accessory muscles, thin, ↑A-P diameter, ↓ chest movement, ↓ diaphragm movement	Normal or ↓ fremitus	Hyper-resonance	↓BS, crackles (all types), wheeze
Large mass	Usually normal	↓ fremitus (AW occluded) ↑ fremitus (if not)	Dull	↓BS (if airway occluded) ↑Bronchial BS (if not) Crackles (fine), rub (maybe)
Pleural effusion	↑ RR, dyspnea, ↓ chest movement (same side), tracheal deviation (opposite side), cyanosis	↓ fremitus	Dull or flat (may be only way to distinguish from a pneumothorax)	↓BS, pleural rub (maybe), egophony (above effusion)

Disease	Inspection	Palpation	Percussion	Auscultation
Pleural thickening	↓ chest movement (same side).	↓ fremitus	Dull	↓BS
Pneumonia	↑RR, dyspnea, cough, ↓ chest movement (same side), pleuritic pain (maybe), cyanosis (maybe), fever	↑ fremitus	Dull	↓BS +/or ↑ bronchial BS, crackles (vary with stage), pleural rub (maybe), bronchophony
Pneumothorax	↑RR, dyspnea, ↓ chest movement and expanded if closed, tracheal deviation (same side, other side if tension), cyanosis	↓ fremitus	Hyper-resonance or tympany	↓BS
Pulmonary edema	↑RR, dyspnea, orthopnea, ↑accessory muscle use, pale or cyanosis	↑ fremitus	Dull	↑ bronchovesicular BS, crackles (medium), wheeze (maybe)
Pulmonary embolism	↑RR, dyspnea, ↑HR, apprehension, cough, sharp chest pain, hemoptysis	Normal	Normal	↓BS (locally), crackles, wheeze, pleural rub (locally)
Pulmonary Interstitial fibrosis	Rapid, shallow breathing, ↑accessory muscle use, dyspnea on exertion, cyanosis (late), clubbing (maybe)	Normal or ↑ fremitus	Normal or dull	↑ bronchovesicular BS (maybe), crackles (fine), whispered pectoriloquy

1-17

Respiratory Physiology Assessment

Assessment of Oxygenation: see Chapter 10

Assessment of Ventilation:

	Norm.	Ab-norm		Norm.	Ab-norm
Adequacy			**Efficiency**		
$\dot{V}_E$	5-7 L/min	↑↓	V_D phys	1/3 $\dot{V}_E$	↑↓
$PaCO_2$	35-45 mmHg	↑↓	V_D/V_T	0.33-0.45	↑↓
$PETCO_2$	35-43 mmHg (4.6 - 5.6%)	↑↓			
$Pa\text{-}ETCO_2$	1-5 mmHg	> 6			

Assessment of Load (ventilatory mechanics)

Adequacy	Normal	Abnormal
Cdyn	40-70 mL/cmH2O	↓
Cstat	70-100 mL/cmH2O	↓
Raw	0.5 - 2.5 cmH2O /L/ sec @ 0.5 L/sec (4-8 with ET tube)	> 15 cmH2O/L/sec
RSBI (f/VT)	<105	>105

Assessment of Capacity (ventilatory mechanics)

	Normal	Abnormal
Adequacy		
Respiratory Drive (P0.1)	< 2 cm H2O	> 4-6 cm H2O
Respiratory Muscle Strength		
VC	60-80 mL/kg	< 60 mL/kg
PImax (MIP, NIF)	< -60 cm H2O	> -30 cmH2O
Respiratory Muscle Endurance		
MVV	120-180 L/min	< 20 L/min
$\dot{V}_E$/MVV	< 1:2	> 1:2

Cardiovascular Assessment

Heart

Inspection/Palpation

PMI-5th left IC space, mid-clavicular line; often ↓ in COPD and shift-
ed down to left sternal border; shifts towards a lobar collapse and
away from a tension pneumothorax; shifts left in cardiomegaly

Pulmonic Area - 2nd left IC space near sternal border, ↑ vibrations
with pulmonary hypertension

Auscultation - Heart sounds

RespiratoryUpdate.com has links to sample sounds

S1	S2
Closure of A-V valves (ventricular contraction), beginning systole, loudest at apex.	Closure of semilunar valves (ventricular relaxation), during diastole, loudest at base. Split may be normal (↑ during I) Split abnormal (width ↑) in pulmonary hypertension or stenosis.

S3	S4
Abnormal rapid vent. filling during diastole, (normal in young, healthy children) Associated with CHF	Active filling of ventricles by atrial contraction (late diastole), may be normal and abnormal

Intensity

Normal = clear sounds

At base of heart: S1 < S2
At apex of heart: S1 > S2

Abnormal ↑ = pulmonary hypertension (S2), cor pulmonale

Abnormal ↓ (distant or muffled) =
heart failure, obesity, pneumothorax,
pulm hyperinflation, valve abnorm.

Abnormal Heart Sounds

Gallop Rhythms	Murmurs	
Ventricular gallop: Abnormal presence of S3 **Atrial gallop:** Abnormal presence of S4	I Barely audible II Audible III Moderately loud IV Loud, no thrill V Very loud, thrill VI Audible off chest	**Systolic:** Incompetent AV or stenotic semilunar **Diastolic:** Incompetent semilunar or stenotic AV

Fluid and Electrolyte Assessment (see also labs chapter)
Urine Output:

Average	1,200 mL / Day	~40 mL / hr
Male	900-1,800 mL/Day	or > 0.5 mL/kg/hr
Female	600-1,600 mL/Day	

Normal Electrolyte Values affecting Ventil. Muscles:

Potassium	K^+	3.5-5.0 mEq/L
Magnesium	Mg^{++}	1.3-2.5 mEq/L
Phosphate	PO^{4-}	1.4-2.7 mEq/L

Fluid Balance Assessment

Fluid Excess	Fluid Deficit
↑body weight, ↑CO, ↑BP ↑PAP, ↑CVP , ↑JVD ↓Hgb, ↓Hct Bounding pulse Moist mucous membranes Pitting edema Pulmonary edema ↑UO from overload ↓UO (< 0.5 mL/kg/hr x 2 hr)	↓body weight, ↓BP(postural) ↑HR, ↓PAP, ↓CVP, ↓JVD ↑Hgb, ↑Hct Poor peripheral pulse Dry mucous membranes Extremities: cool/pale & trunk: warm/dry, ↓skin elasticity ↑UO (diuresis) ↓ capillary refill

Changes in Fluid Balance - Causes of

↑Fluid (Hypervolemia)		↓Fluid (Hypovolemia)	
↑Intake	↓Output		
Iatrogenic	↓**Renal Perfusion:** Heart Failure PPV (↓CO, ↑ADH) Renal System Malfunction Blocked Foley	Dehydration Starvation **Fluid Shift:** Burns, Shock	Burns Diarrhea Diuresis Hemorrhage Vomiting

Neurological Assessment

Vital Signs	RR, HR, BP
Motor Activity	Ability to cough/clear secretions Grip strength Motions: coordination, paralysis, tremors Ability to follow commands Positions: <u>Decorticate</u> – flexed arms, hands fisted extended legs, plantar flexion <u>Decerebrate</u> - extended arms, extended legs, plantar flexion Pupil size and reaction
Mental Status	Emotional state, behavior, comfort, orientation LOC – See below

Modified Glasgow Coma Scale
Scale from 3 (comatose) to 15 (fully alert)

Adult/Older Children	Score	Infant/Young Children
Eye Opening		
Spontaneous	4	Spontaneous
To speech	3	To loud noise
To pain	2	To pain
Not at all	1	Not at all
Verbal Response		
Oriented	5	Smiles, coos, cries appropriately
Confused	4	Irritable and cries
Inappropriate	3	Inappropriate crying
Incomprehensible	2	Grunts and moans
None	1	None
Motor Response		
Obeys commands	6	Spontaneous movement
Localizes pain	5	Withdraws to touch
Withdraws from pain	4	Withdraws from pain
Flexion to pain	3	Flexion to pain
Extension to pain	2	Extension to pain
None	1	None

Descriptive Terms for Level of Consciousness (LOC)

Alert	Awake, oriented and responds appropriately
Confused	Inability to think clearly impaired judgment
Disoriented	Starting loss of consciousness disoriented to time/place
Lethargic	Sleepy, arouses easily, responds appropriately
Obtunded	Awakens only with difficulty, then responds appropriately
Stuporous	Does not completely awaken Responds only to deep pain Withdraws or pushes you away
Unresponsive	Responds only to deep pain, exhibits reflex
Comatose	No response, flaccid muscle tone

2   Arterial Blood Gases

The Oxygenation Aspect of ABGs is covered in
Chapter 10: Respiratory Procedures

Oakes' ABG Pocket Guide/Instruction Guide Set is a comprehensive resource for understanding ABG classification and analysis.

It can be purchased at **RespiratoryBooks.com**

Normal Parameters	Arterial		Mixed Venous	
	Norm	Range	Norm	Range
pH (pHa, pH$\overline{v}$), units	7.40	7.35-7.45	7.36	7.31-7.41
PCO$_2$ (PaCO$_2$, P$\overline{v}$CO$_2$), mmHg	40	35-45	46	41-51
PO$_2$ (PaO$_2$, P$\overline{v}$O$_2$), mmHg*	100	80-100	40	35-42
O$_2$ Sat (SaO$_2$, S$\overline{v}$O$_2$), %	97%	95-100%	75%	68-77%
HCO$_3$, mEq/L	24	22-26	24	22-26
TCO$_2$	25	23-27	25	23-27
BE, mEq/L	0	+/- 2	0	+/- 2
O$_2$ content (CaO$_2$, C$\overline{v}$O$_2$), mL/dL	20	15-24	15	12-15

*21% at sea level

Sampling for Arterial Blood Gas Analysis[1,2]

Indications

Need to evaluate:
Oxygenation (PaO2, SaO2, HbO2, Hgb total, dyshemoglobins)
Ventilation (PaCO2)
Acid-base (pH, PaCO2)
Need to quantitate patient's response to: therapy and/or diagnostic evaluation.
Monitor disease severity and progression.

Contraindications

Hand puncture – negative Allen test
Any limb site – infection, PVD, surgical shunt
Femoral puncture –outside the hospital
Coagulopathy or anticoagu lant therapy (relative)

Hazards/Complications

Anaphylaxis (local anesthetic)
Arterial occlusion
Arteriospasm
Contagion at site
Emboli (air or blood)
Hematoma
Hemorrhage
Pain
Trauma to vessel
Vasovagal response

Monitoring

Patient: RR, temperature, clinical appearance, position and/or activity level, puncture site (post sample).
O2/vent therapy: proper application of O2 device , FIO2 or flowrate, ventilator mode and settings.
Procedure: ease or difficulty, pulsatile blood return, air bubbles or clot.

Frequency

Dependent on clinical status and indication, alternate sites or A-line is indicated for multiple sampling.

Clinical Goals

(desired outcome)
Sample obtained without contamination from: air, anticoagulant, flush solution, or venous blood.
Sample obtained without clotting from: improper anticoagulant, improper mixing, or air exposure.

---

1) ABG sampling is blood drawn, via puncture or A-line, from a peripheral artery to measure PaO2, PaCO2, pH, Hgb total, CoHgb, and/or MetHgb.
2) Adapted from AARC Clinical Practice Guideline: Sampling for Arterial Blood Gas Analysis, *Respiratory Care*, Volume 37, #8, 1992

ABG INTERPRETATION =

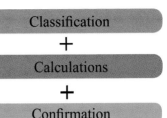

Classification

+

Calculations

+

Confirmation

A. Classification

Respiratory
Acidosis   Alkalosis

Metabolic
Acidosis   Alkalosis

B. Calculations

Calculate Compensation and Gaps:
Determines whether or not the body is compensating and whether or not other primary disorders exist.
Determine Oxygenation Status

C. Confirmation

Consistency with patient assessment, patient's baseline and check for accuracy: Determines validity of Classification and Calculations

KEYS to INTERPRETATION

1. Initial Technical Classification DOES NOT always equal a definitive ABG interpretation
2. Calculations are always ESSENTIAL
3. Patient assessment is ESSENTIAL
4. Patient BASELINE VALUES are often invaluable
5. Always check for POSSIBLE INACCURACIES in the gas result
6. SERIAL ABGs are often more important than a single ABG
7. ABG interpretation often leads to LIFE and DEATH decisions. Obviously errors are unacceptable!

STEPS OF ABG INTERPRETATION

A) Classification (see chart next page)

Primary Problem
Step 1. Check pH – Acidosis or Alkalosis?

Primary Cause
Step 2. Check PaCO2 – is Respiratory the primary cause?

Step 3. Check HCO_3^- – is Metabolic the primary cause?

Compensation
Step 4. Is the body compensating?

Initial Classification
Step 5. Technical Classification and/or Functional Classification

B) Calculations

Step 6. Determine if Compensation is Appropriate or are there other Primary Disorders

	PaCO₂	pH	HCO₃
Respiratory Acidosis			
Acute	↑ 10	↓ 0.08	↑ 1
Chronic	↑ 10	↓ 0.03	↑ 4
Respiratory Alkalosis			
Acute	↓ 10	↑ 0.08	↓ 2
Chronic	↓ 10	↑ 0.03	↓ 5

	HCO₃	pH	PaCO₂
Metabolic Acidosis	↓ 1	↓ 0.015	↓ 1.2
Metabolic Alkalosis	↑ 1	↑ 0.015	↑ 0.7

Step 7. Determine Anion Gap and Bicarbonate Gap

a. Anion Gap: $AG = Na - (Cl + HCO_3)$

b. Bicarbonate Gap (if an AG acidosis):

$BG = $ Patient's $HCO_3 + \Delta\ AG$

BG Norm = 24 = AG Metabolic Acidosis

< 20 = AG Met. Acidosis + Non AG Met. Acidosis

> 28 = AG Met. Acidosis + Met. Alkalosis

Step 8. Determine Oxygenation

C) Confirmation

Step 9.   Systematically Assess Patient

Step 10. Check for Accuracy (errors)

Step 11. **Final Interpretations**

| | Primary Cause | | | | Compensation | Initial Classification |
| Primary Problem | | Primary Cause | | | | |
Step 1: Check pH	Step 2: Check PaCO2 (35-45)	Step 2: Is Respiratory 1°?	Step 3: Check HCO3 (22-26)	Step 3: Is Metabolic 1°?	Step 4: Is the body compensating? (Yes/No)	Step 5: Technical Classification (1)
	↑		↑	Yes	Yes (↑ PaCO2)	PC Metabolic Alkalosis
	N		↑	Yes	-	Metabolic Alkalosis (UC)
Alkalosis > 7.45*	↓	Yes	↑	Yes	-	Mixed Respiratory Alkalosis & Metabolic Alkalosis
	↓	Yes	N,↓		(3)	Respiratory Alkalosis (UC)
	↓	Yes	↓		Yes (↓ HCO3)	PC Respiratory Alkalosis
	↑	Yes or compensat.?	↑	Yes or compensat?	Yes (↑ PaCO2)	FC Metabolic Alkalosis (7.41 - 7.45)
			↑		Yes (↑ HCO3)	FC Respiratory Acidosis (7.35-7.39)
Normal 7.35-7.45	N		N		-	Normal or Mixed Disorder (2)
	↓	Yes or compensating?	↓	Yes or compensating?	Yes (↓ PaCO2)	FC Metabolic Acidosis (7.35-7.39)
			↓		Yes (↓ HCO3)	FC Respiratory Alkalosis (7.41-7.45)

↑	Yes	↑		Yes (↑ HCO$_3$)	PC Respiratory Acidosis
↑	Yes	N, ↑		(3)	Respiratory Acidosis (UC)
↑	Yes	↓	Yes	-	Mixed Respiratory & Metabolic Acidosis
N		↓	Yes	-	Metabolic Acidosis (UC)
↓		↓	Yes	Yes (↓ PaCO2)	PC Metabolic Acidosis

Acidosis < 7.35 **

(1) Technical classification terminology:

    UC = Uncompensated (no compensation has occurred). Common usage leaves this designation off.

    PC = Partially Compensated (pH has returned part way back to normal range)

    FC = Fully Compensated (pH has returned back to normal range)

(2) Mixed Disorder (opposite disorders) = Respiratory acidosis & metabolic alkalosis or respiratory alkalosis & metabolic acidosis

    (PaCO$_2$ and HCO$_3$ go in same direction and "apparent compensation" is greater than expected)

(3) The immediate change in HCO$_3$ from normal is due to the hydrolysis effect, rather than compensation.

* As pH moves towards 7.8 = ↑ CNS stimulation: irritability, arrhythmias, tetany, convulsions, respiratory arrest, death.
Definitive therapy is indicated at pH > 7.6.

** As pH moves towards 7.0 = ↓ CNS stimulation: drowsiness, lethargy, coma, death. Definitive therapy is often considered at pH < 7.15.

2-6

ABG Disorders

Technical Class.	Functional Class.	Compensation Status
UC Respiratory Acidosis	Acute Respiratory Acidosis	**Kidneys:** Either not enough time to begin compensation or the kidneys are compromised
PC Respiratory Acidosis	Chronic Respiratory Acidosis	**Kidneys:** Either not enough time to fully compensate or compensation is maximal (chronic), but pH not back to normal range
FC Respiratory Acidosis	Chronic Respiratory Acidosis	**Kidneys:** Compensation is maximal (chronic) and full – pH is back to normal range (occurs only in very mild disorders)
UC Respiratory Alkalosis	Acute Respiratory Alkalosis	**Kidneys:** Either not enough time to begin compensation or kidneys are compromised
PC Respiratory Alkalosis	Chronic Respiratory Alkalosis	**Kidneys:** Either not enough time to fully compensate or compensation is maximal (chronic), but pH not back to normal range
FC Respiratory Alkalosis	Chronic Respiratory Alkalosis	**Kidneys:** Compensation is maximal (chronic) and full –pH is back to normal range (occurs in most disorders)
UC Metabolic Acidosis	Metabolic Acidosis*	**Respiratory:** system is compromised (rare that there is zero compensation) or such a mild change in HCO$_3$ that any change in PaCO$_2$ is minimal.
PC Metabolic Acidosis	Metabolic Acidosis	**Respiratory:** Compensation is usually immediate and maximal, but pH is not back to normal range
FC Metabolic Acidosis	Metabolic Acidosis	**Respiratory:** This classification essentially *does not exist* because PaCO2 generally does not return pH back to normal range. If pH is normal, there is usually a secondary respiratory disorder at work.
UC Metabolic Alkalosis	Metabolic Alkalosis	**Respiratory:** If there is no compensation, there is usually a secondary respiratory alkalosis
PC Metabolic Alkalosis	Metabolic Alkalosis	**Respiratory:** Compensation is usually immediate and maximal, but pH is not back to normal range
FC Metabolic Alkalosis	Metabolic Alkalosis	**Respiratory:** This class. really *does not exist* because PaCO2 generally does not return pH back to normal range. If pH is normal, there is usually a secondary respiratory disorder at work.

NOTES

Technical classification terminology:

UC = Uncompensated (no compensation has occurred). Common usage leaves this designation off.

PC = Partially Compensated (pH has returned part way back to normal range)

FC = Fully Compensated (pH has returned back to normal range)

A *corrected* blood gas disorder is one in which the pH is returned to normal range by altering the component primarily affected.

A *compensated* blood gas disorder is one in which the pH is returned towards normal range by altering the component not primarily affected.

Because of the limitations of the lungs or kidneys to "fully" compensate for most alterations of each other (i.e., completely return pH to normal), "full" or "complete" compensation is more appropriately referred to as "*maximal*" compensation.

Maximal Compensation = the body has completely compensated all it is designed to compensate – usually pH returns only 50% of the way back.

If the disorder is *mild*, maximal compensation may return the pH to within normal range, resulting in a "*full*" compensation (FC).

If the disorder is *moderate* to *severe*, maximal compensation will only return the pH part way back to normal range, resulting in a "*partial*" compensation (PC).

* The terms "*acute*" and "*chronic*" for metabolic disorders are often omitted because, *functionally*, there is usually no time distinction between acute and chronic metabolic disorders – the respiratory system compensation is usually immediate. Also, because all metabolic disorders are essentially Partially Compensated, all metabolic disorders are simply termed Metabolic Acidosis or Metabolic Alkalosis, without any further descriptive terminology.

See Equation Chapter for a Complete List of Acid-Base Equations

See Respiratory Procedures, Chapter 10 for extensive Oxygenation information, including assessment, interpretation, devices, and more.

ABG Accuracy Check

1. ***Check Patient – Does ABG line up with patient's clinical condition?***
   Good gases & patient in distress; Bad gases & no patient distress?
   Rising or normal PaCO2 in severe respiratory distress (e.g., asthma)?

2. ***Check Lab Values***

   HCO_3 should be within 1-2 mEq/L of Total CO_2
   A difference of > 4 mEq/L = technical error

   Actual HCO_3 should = 24 x PaCO2/ (80 - last two digits of pH)
   (only works for pH between 7.30 – 7.50)

3. ***Check for Errors***
   A) Sampling Errors
   1) Venous blood or contamination with venous blood ($\downarrow$ PaO2,
      $\uparrow$ PaCO2, $\downarrow$ pH).
      Venous PaO2 ≈ 40 (or does not match patient clinical
      condition; cross check with SpO2)
   2) Air in sample – Effect varies with agitation, duration, temp, &
      volume.
      (PaO2 higher than expected; PaCO2 lower than expected)

Air		Blood
O_2 159 mmHg	→	↑ PaO2 (unless > 159)
CO_2 0 mmHg	→	↓ PaCO2 → ↑ pH

   This can result in a negative PA-aO2!
   3) Anticoagulant (heparin) - too much (rare today, but same
      effect as air).
   4) Patient not on reported FIO2
   5) Patient not in a steady state (ABG too soon after a change in
      FIO2 or MV)

   B) Measuring Errors
   1) Improper calibration, quality control, or sample mixing
   2) Documentation/transcription errors (PaCO2/PaO2 reversed?
      orally conveyed?)
   3) Wrong patient's blood
   4) Time delay in measuring (> 30 min. un-iced; > 60 min. iced)
   5) ↑ WBC or platelets → ↓ PaO2 (leukocyte larceny)

4. ***Check PaO2 – FIO2 Relationship***
   A) On room air: PaO2 should be < 130 mmHg
   B) On ↑ FIO2: PaO2 should be < 5 x FIO2
      (Example: FIO2 0.4; PaO2 should be < 200)
   C) Always question: Was mask on patient, cannula in nose, etc.?

5. ***Check PaO2/SaO2 – SpO2 relationship (See page 10-76)***

3 Chest X-Ray (CXR) Interpretation

Keys to Good CXR Interpretation

1. **Be Systematic.**
   Regardless of the system you adopt, review every CXR in the same order, every time. Otherwise, you may miss something critical. We present our systematic approach on pg 3-2.

2. **Be Aware.**
   The CXR must be interpreted in context of the patient's status. Avoid treating an X-Ray, "just because it looks bad," but use it as another tool.

3. **Be Wary.**
   Use caution in making decisions (such as pulling back an Endotracheal Tube) based solely upon a CXR. Body habitus, poor quality, and other factors can make locating tubes difficult at times.

Systematic Approach to Interpreting a CXR

see also: Abnormal Appearances on pg 3-5

1. **Confirm patient.**
2. **Confirm date and time.**
3. **Identify type:** AP or PA (special: lateral decubitis)
4. **Check quality:** about 4 vertebrae visible, Inspiratory Film?
   Exp film may show abnorm ↑ heart size, ↓ volume, ↑ interstitium
5. **Check rotation:** clavicles centered around vertebrae
6. **Systematically explore from Outside-to-Inside:**

<table>
<tr><td>Soft Tissue</td><td>Amount of tissue (obesity, breasts)
Subcutaneous emphysema (crepitus)</td></tr>
<tr><td>Bones</td><td>Examine for fractures, especially clavicles, ribs.
Obvious spinal deformity (kyphosis, etc.)?</td></tr>
<tr><td>Heart</td><td>Size: > 60% of thoracic width = abnormal[1]
Identify: Major structures (ventricles, etc.)</td></tr>
<tr><td>Lungs</td><td>Expansion (7-9 ribs, mid-clavic. at diaphragm)
Find trachea, carina (midline?)
Find fissures, if visible
Find hila (L is above R)
Costophrenic and Cardiophrenic Angles
   (blunted ~fluid?)
Diaphragm: Right is slightly ↑ than Left (liver)
               Elevated? Flattened (air trap)?
Parenchyma:
   Haziness (~atelctasis)
   Consolidation (air bronchograms at periphery)
   Infiltrates (consolidation, localized or diffuse)
   Pneumothorax (lack of vasc. markings)
   General abnormalities (foreign objects,
              nodules, honeycombing, etc.)</td></tr>
<tr><td>Tubes Lines</td><td>ET Tube (3-5 cm above carina)
Trach Tube (present or not)
Gastric tube
Chest tube(s)
EKG leads
Central Line / Pulmonary Artery Line</td></tr>
</table>

[1]Be careful when interpreting heart size with AP films (typical of critical care) which may over-estimate size.

Normal Chest X-Ray (CXR) - Posterior-Anterior

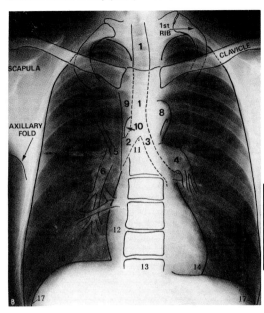

1. trachea
2. right mainstem
3. left mainstem
4. left pulmonary artery
5. right upper lobe pulmonary vein
6. right interlobar artery
7. right upper and lower lobe vein
8. aortic knob
9. superior vena cava
10. ascending aorta
11. carina
12. right atrium
13. right ventricle
14. left ventricle
15. left hemidiaphragm
16. right hemidiaphragm
17. costophrenic angle
18. minor fissure

Normal Chest X-Ray (CXR) - Lateral

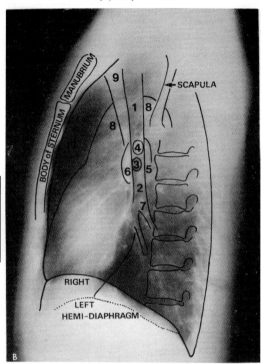

1. trachea
2. right intermediate bronchus
3. left upper lobe bronchus
4. right upper lobe bronchus
5. left interlobar artery
6. right interlobar artery
7. pulmonary veins
8. aortic arch
9. brachiocephalic vessels
10. substernal space

Reprinted with permission from Fraser, R.H. and Pare, J.A.: *Organ Physiology: Structure and Function of the Lung*. Copyright 1977 by W.B Saunders, Co., Philadelphia

Abnormal Appearances and Possible Causes

Appearances	Possible Causes
Air Bronchogram – Can visualize airways out towards the periphery	Usually occurs with consolidated alveoli
AP vs. PA Projection – AP usually shows ↓ lung volumes, elevated hemi-diaphragms, ↑ lung marking in bases, heart enlarged, scapula overlies upper fields, often rotated	Portable x-ray, AP usually taken for bed-ridden patients (esp. while on MV)
Butterfly Pattern:	
Puffy cloudiness in central lung fields	Pulmonary edema
Honeycomb cloudiness throughout lung fields	Interstitial edema
Costophrenic Blunting – Rounded angle	Fluid in pleural space
↑ Heart Size:	
RV – Pulmonary artery pushed towards L cardiac border	Cor pulmonale
RA	Cor pulmonale
LV – Rounding of L cardiac border and boot-shaped extension	CHF
LA – Lateral projection of R cardiac border	CHF
Kerley B Lines – Perpendicular lines to pleura in peripheral bases	Interstitial edema
Miliary Pattern – Small, round regular densities	Alveolar filling with fluid or material
Nodular Pattern – Confluent densities of different sizes	↑ Interstitial or alveolar pattern
↓ Peripheral Markings – ↓ or absent markings in periphery	Air in pleural space, pulmonary hypertension, pulmonary embolism
Dilated Pulmonary Arteries – Antler-shaped, cloudiness at base	Pulmonary hypertension
Reticular Pattern – Irregular network of straight or curved densities	Interstitial infiltrates or fibrosis
Reticulogranular Pattern – Ground glass appearance	ARDS

Silhouette Sign – Loss of the normal silhouette of the heart, aorta, or diaphragm (*See below*)	Water density (infiltrates) in anatomic contact with heart, aorta, or diaphragm
Volume ↓ – ↓ Size of thoracic cage, elevated diaphragms, ↑ interstitial markings	Atelectasis, ↓ surfactant, ↓ CL
Volume ↑ – ↑ size of thoracic cage (hyper-aeration), flattened diaphragm, ↓ interstitial markings	*Trapped air:* asthma, emphysema, ↑MV volumes, ↑ PEEP or auto-PEEP, tension pneumothorax

*See Chapter 11 for X-ray appearance of specific diseases and disorders

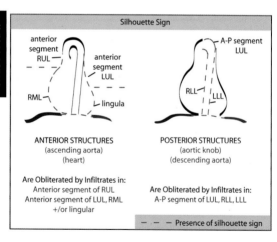

Silhouette Sign

anterior segment RUL
anterior segment LUL
RML
lingula

A-P segment LUL
RLL
LLL

ANTERIOR STRUCTURES
(ascending aorta)
(heart)

Are Obliterated by Infiltrates in:
Anterior segment of RUL
Anterior segment of LUL, RML
+/or lingular

POSTERIOR STRUCTURES
(aortic knob)
(descending aorta)

Are Obliterated by Infiltrates in:
A-P segment of LUL, RLL, LLL

– – – Presence of silhouette sign

Segmental Infiltrates on the Chest X-Ray (CXR)

This diagram shows the relative location of infiltrates as they appear on a Chest X-Ray (CXR). Knowing this may aid in positioning for postural drainage.

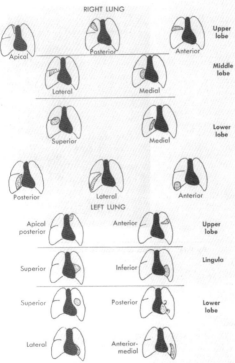

Reprinted with permission from Sheldon, R.L..In Scanlan, C.L., Spearman, C.B. and Sheldon, R.L., editors: *Egan's Fundamentals of Respiratory Therapy*, 6th ed. Copyright 1995 by the Mosby Yearbook, Inc., St. Louis

Common Chest X-Ray Findings by Disease/Disorder -
See individual disease/disorder in Disease Chapter

Approximate Tube/Line Placement on CXR

Line/Tube	Placement
Endotracheal Tube	Tip should be midline 2-6 cm above carina (adult)
Tracheostomy Tube	Tip should be midline 1/2 to 1/3 distance between stoma/carina
CVP Line	Tip should be in Superior Vena Cava, just before Right Atrium
PA Catheter	Tip should in right or left Pulmonary Artery (about 5 cm distal to main pulmonary artery bifurcation)
NG or OG Tube	Tip and side hole should be beyond gastroesophageal junction
Chest Tube	Tip of Radiopaque line should be within the pleural space and medial to the inner margin of the ribs Positioning depends on whether collecting air or fluid

Verify Tube or Line placement in multiple
ways - do not rely solely on the CXR.

4 ECG Interpretation

How To Read An ECG

1. Check for calibration (10mm high box with strip moving 25 mm/sec) and assess for artifact.
2. Measure ventricular rate (See below)
3. Check P wave (Shape, position, and # = atrial rate)
4. Measure P-R interval (Normal = 0.12 - 0.20 seconds)
5. Evaluate QRS shape and interval (Normal < 0.12 seconds)
6. Check regularity of waves (the distance between R-R waves should not vary > 0.12 seconds)
7. Evaluate T wave and ST segment (See Pg 4-10)

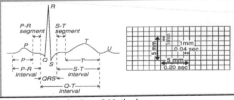

Measuring Ventricular Rate: 2 Methods

1. **Irregular rhythms (or slow)**: Count # R waves (in 6 seconds; i.e., two 3 sec intervals or 2 boxes) X 10 = rate/min
2. **Regular Rhythms**: "Rule of 300": Count # of large boxes between R waves (start with 1 on a red line). Divide 300 by the # of boxes.

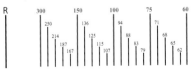

ECGs

Standard ECG Leads

Limb		Chest		
Positive Electrode				
I	Left arm	V1	R of sternum in 4th ICS	
II	Left leg	V2	L of sternum in 4th ICS	
III	Left leg	V3	Midway between V2 and V4	
aVR	Right arm	V4	Midclavicular line in 5th ICS	
aVL	Left arm	V5	Anterior axillary, same level as V4	
aVF	Left leg	V6	Midaxillary line, same level as V4	
Negative Electrode				

Negative Electrode		**Problem in:**	**Check Leads:**
I	Right arm	V1-V6	Chest lead that corresponds to tracing
II	Right arm	Lead I	LA, RA
III	Left arm	Lead II	LL, RA
		Lead III	LL, LA
TROUBLESHOOTING		aVR	RA, LA, LL
		aVL	LA, RA, LL
		aVF	LL, RA, LA

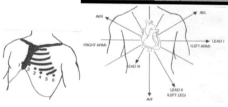

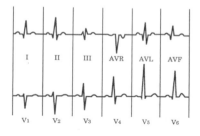

4-2

Interpreting ECGs: According to Rate

Normal	Slow	Fast
Sinus rhythm	Sinus bradycardia	Sinus tachycardia
Sinus arrhythmia	(< 60/min)	(>100/min)
SA block	AV nodal rhythm	PAT (150-250)
Wandering	(40-60/min)	Atrial flutter
pacemaker	2nd ° AV block	(250-350)
PAC	(1/2 to 1/3 atrial rate)	Atrial fib (350-450)
PNC	3rd ° AV block	AV nodal tach
1st ° AV block	(< 40/min)	(150-250)
PVC	V-fib / V standstill (0/min)	V-tach (150-250)

According to P Wave

	Absent	Buried	Abnormal	Inverted
Wandering pacemaker		X	X	
PAC			X	X
PAT		X	X	
Atrial Flutter			X	
A-fib	X		X	
PNC		X		X
AV nodal tachycardia		X		X
AV nodal rhythm		X		X
PVC	X			
V-tach	X			

According to Prolonged PR Intervals

P with every QRS	1st ° Heart Block
Progressive PR prolongation	2nd ° Heart Block (Type I)
Constant PR with dropped beats	2nd ° Heart Block (Type II)
No relation between P and QRS	3rd ° Heart Block

Classification of Cardiac Arrhythmias (by Prognosis)

Minor Arrhythmias	Major Arrhythmias	
Sinus Tachycardia	PAC (> 6/min)	Sinoatrial Arrest
Sinus Bradycardia	Atrial Tachycardia	1st ° Heart Block
Sinus Arrhythmia	Atrial Flutter	2nd ° Heart Block
PAC (< 6/min)	Atrial Fibrillation	3rd ° Heart Block
PVC (< 6/min)	PVC (> 6/min)	Bundle Branch Block
PNC (< 6/min)	AV Nodal Rhythm	
Wandering Pacemaker		

Death Producing: Ventricular Tachycardia / Fibrillation / Standstill

ECGs

Summary of Basic Arrhythmias (according to site of origin)

Type	Identifying Features	Appearance (Lead II)	Clinical Notes
SA Node			
Normal Sinus Rhythm	Rate: 60-100/min, P waves regular P-R Interval (0.12-0.20), QRS regular (< 0.12), R-R regular, T wave upright and round, ST segment is flat		Normal Rhythm
Sinus Arrhythmia	↓ R-R interval on inspiration, irregular rhythm		Probably vagal stimulation from pressures in thorax, benign, no Tx needed
Sinus Tachycardia	Rate > 100/min		Causes – Fever, hypoxemia, ↓BP, hypovolemia, pain, sepsis, heart failure, bronchodilators. May lead to ischemia.
Sinus Bradycardia	Rate < 60/min		Causes – Carotid massage, hypothermia, Valsalva, tracheal Sx. May lead to ↓BP/CO, syncope, CHF, shock. Note some athletes have a resting HR < 60
Sinus (SA) Block (arrest)	Entire beat absent		Also called Sino-atrial arrest or escape.
Wandering Pacemaker	Rate varies, P waves vary in shape & position, P-R interval varies		Rate >100 = Multifocal Atrial Tachycardia (MAT). Seen in COPD or digitalis toxicity.

Type	Identifying Features	Appearance (Lead II)	Clinical Notes
Atrial			
Premature Atrial Contractions (PAC)	Premature P waves (abnormal or inverted), short T-P interval before beat, long T-P after beat		May confuse with Premature Nodal Contraction.
Premature Atrial Tachycardia (PAT, PSVT)	Rate 150-250/min, P waves abnormal or buried. Called supraventricular tach (SVT) and may be paroxysmal.		Sudden onset and termination. Patients may experience lightheadedness or palpitations. May lead to ↓BP/CO, myocardial ischemia, CHF.
Atrial Flutter	Atrial rate 250-350/min, ventricular rate normal, sawtooth P waves, 2:1, 3:1, 4:1 block of QRS		Commonly associated with pulmonary disease. May return to normal or deteriorate to A-fib. ↑ risk for embolism.
Atrial Fibrillation (A-fib)	No clear P waves, atrial rate 350-450/min, irregular ventricular rhythm		Often asymptomatic, except ↓ cardiac reserve. ↑ risk for embolism.
Nodal			
Premature Nodal Contractions	P wave absent or inverted after the QRS		PJC (or PNC) — Premature junctional complex May confuse with PAC

ECGs

4-5

Type	Identifying Features	Appearance (Lead II)	Clinical Notes
Paroxysmal Junctional (A-V nodal) Tachycardia	Rate 150-250/min, P wave variable		
A-V Nodal (Junctional) Rhythm	Rate 40-60/min, P waves absent or inverted		Also called junctional escape or idiojunctional rhythm.
1st ° A-V Heart Block	Constant, prolonged P-R interval (> 0.2 sec)		Often asymptomatic. May be misread as a normal sinus rhythm
2nd ° A-V Heart Block (Type I, Wenckebach)	Progressively longer P-R interval until a beat is dropped		Often asymptomatic
2nd ° A-V Heart Block (Type II)	Some non-conducted P waves (no QRS), constant P-R intervals, slow ventricular rate		May lead to ↓ BP/CO, weakness, and fainting. Also called Mobitz II
3rd ° A-V Heart Block (Complete)	No relationship between P waves and QRS, atrial rate normal		Atria and ventricles beat independently (A-V dissociation). Rate 40 – 60/min = Junctional rhythm Rate < 40/min = Ventricular rhythm

Type	Identifying Features	Appearance (Lead II)	Clinical Notes
Bundle Branch Block (R or L)	QRS widened (>/= 0.12) with rabbit-ear feature		Appearance highly variable Cause: underlying heart disease
Ventricular			
Premature Ventricular Contractions (PVC)	Premature, wide (> 0.12), distorted QRS with no P wave, T wave opposite, full compensatory pause		> 6/min is pathological. Most common cause is myocardial ischemia. May be caused by anxiety, ↓K+, excessive caffeine, or medications. R-on-T may lead to V-tach.
Bigeminy = 1 normal coupled with 1 PVC Trigeminy = 2 normal coupled with 1 PVC		Couplet = 2 PVCs side by side Triplet = 3 PVCs in a row	
Unifocal = 2 or more PVCs that look alike (same heart site) Multifocal = 2 or more PVCs that look different (different sites)			
Ventricular Tachycardia (V-Tach*)	Series of PVCs (> 3 in row) rate 150-250/min		May quickly lead to ↓BP/CO, V-fib, loss of consciousness, and death.
Ventricular Flutter	Series of smooth sine waves, rate 250-350/min		May quickly lead to ↓BP/CO, V-fib, loss of consciousness, and death.

ECGs

4-7

Type	Identifying Features	Appearance (Lead II)	Clinical Notes
Torsades de Pointes	a form of VTach where QRS complex varies beat-to-beat. May change from + to - axis.		May return to NSR or become more serious. Treat with ACLS algorithm for VTach.
Ventricular Fibrillation (V-fib) *	No well defined, erratic QRS, rate 350-450/min		Rhythm may be mistaken for either V-tach or asystole. Immediate ↓CO →coma. Treat with defibrillation.
Ventricular Standstill (Asystole) *	Essentially a flat line		Caution: a simple disconnect of ECG lead can resemble asystole. Check for immediate pulselessness, ↓ BP, and loss of consciousness.
Pulseless Electrical Activity (PEA)	Any heart rhythm that should be producing a palpable pulse, but is not.	Appearance varies: Treat underlying cause H (hypovolemia, hypoxia, ion) (hyperkalemia, hypothermia) O (drug overdose) T (tamponade, tension pneumothorax, thrombosis) Most Common: may follow failure due to hypoxia	

ECG's must be interpreted in light of the patient's clinical symptoms, physical exam, medications, electrolyte balance, body size, and age. Interpretation should not be made solely on the basis of the ECG findings.

4-8

Interpreting Abnormalities *

Pulmonary Effects

COPD	Pulmonary Embolism (→ Cor Pulmonale)
Low voltage in all leads, Rt. axis deviation, MAT	S1Q3⊥3 = Wide S in I, large Q in III, inverted T in III and V1-V4. ST depressed in II, often transient RBBB

Cardiac Hypertrophy

Atrial Hypertrophy: P waves more than 3 small squares wide		
Right Atrial		**Left Atrial**
In VI - Large, diphasic P wave with tall initial component	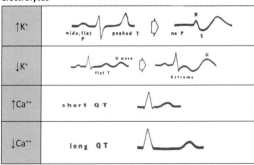	In VI - Large diphasic P wave with wide terminal component
Ventricular Hypertrophy		
Right Ventricular		**Left Ventricular**
R wave > S wave(VI) R wave progressively smaller (VI→ V6). S wave persists in V5 and V6. Wide QRS and right axis deviation		S wave (VI) + R wave (V5) = > 35 mm L axis deviat., wide QRS T wave slants down slowly and returns up rapidly (inverted) (V5 or 6)

Electrolytes

↑K⁺	wide, flat P / peaked T	no P / R S
↓K⁺	U wave / flat T	U / Extreme
↑Ca⁺⁺	short Q-T	
↓Ca⁺⁺	long QT	

Cardiac Ischemia, Injury or Infarction

Acute

Ischemia = Inverted T Wave

Inverted T wave is symmetrical (V2-V6).
Signifies an acute process and usually lasts only a few hours.

Injury = Elevated ST segment

Signifies an acute process and usually lasts only a few hours. If T wave is also elevated off baseline, suspect pericarditis. Location of injury may be determined like infarct location.
ST depression = digitalis, subendocardial infarct or exercise stress test.

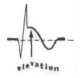

elevation

Acute or Chronic

Infarction = Q Wave

Insignificant (small) Q waves may be normal (esp. V5 and V6).
Significant (abnormal) Q waves must be > one small square (0.04sec) wide or > 1/3 QRS height in lead III.

Q

Location of Infarct (or injury)

Anterior	Q wave in V1,V2,V3 or V4 (ST elevation)
Inferior	Q in II, III, and aVF
Lateral	Q in I and aVL
Posterior	Large R in V1 and V2 (ST depression) Mirror test

ECGs

5 | Laboratory Tests

Selected tests related to Respiratory are presented on the following pages each with commonly used values. Normal values are variable between institutions and the method used, and values of healthy vs. diseased patients may overlap. Drugs and iatrogenic factors are not listed as causes of abnormal values, but should always be considered.

Danger Levels

Electrolytes	Low	High
Na+	< 120 mEq/L	> 160 mEq/L
K+	< 2.5 mEq/L	> 6.5 mEq/L
Hematology		
Hematocrit	< 14%	> 60%
WBC	< 2000 uL	> 50,000 uL
Platelets	< 20,000 uL	> 1,00,000 uL
PT	> 40 sec	
Blood & Serum		
pH	< 7.20	> 7.60
$PaCO_2$	< 20 mmHg	> 60 mmHg
PaO_2	< 40 mmHg	> 100 mmHg (newborn)
HCO_3	< 10 mEq/L	> 40 mEq/L
Glucose	< 40 mg/dL	> 400 mg/dL

LABS

Electrolytes

Test	Normal Value	Clinical Significance	Clinical Increases	Clinical Decreases
Na+ Sodium	135-145 mEq/L SI 135-145 mmol/L	Major extracellular cation, comprises majority of osmotically active solute. Greatly affects distribution of body water.	↑ Na+ – Cushings syndrome, hyperadrenocorticism, excessive intake. ↓Body H2O – Dehydration, hyperpnea, diabetes, diuretics, cardiac failure. S & S – Thirst, viscous mucous, dry, rough tongue.	↓Na+ (with ↓body H2O) – adrenal insufficiency, alkali, burns, diuretics, dehydration, trauma. ↑ renal output, ↓ artificial hyperglycemia, CHF, cirrhosis, inappropriate ADH, renal insufficiency. S & S – ↑ HR, ↓ BP, cold, clammy skin, apprehension, convulsions.
K+ Potassium	3.5-5.0 mEq/L SI 3.5-5.0 mmol/L	Major intracellular cation, maintains intracellular osmolality, affects muscle contraction, plays role in nerve impulses, enzyme action, cell membrane function.	Excessive administration Shift from cells – Acidosis (metabolic), infection, succinylcholine, trauma. ↓ renal output S&S – Arrhythmias; muscle weakness.	Shift into cells – Alkalosis GI loss – anorexia, diarrhea, NG Sx, vomiting. ↑ renal output – Cushings syndrome, diabetic ketoacidosis, diuretics, renal tubular-acidosis, steroid therapy. S&S – Arrhythmias, muscle weak
Cl- Chloride	95-105 mEq/L SI 95-105 mmol/L	Principle extracellular anion, important in acid-base balance	Cardiac decompensation, renal insufficiency, salt intake	COPD, Cushings syndrome, dehydration, diabetic ketoacidosis, diuretics, fever, metab acidosis, pneumonia

Test	Normal Value	Clinical Significance	Clinical Increases	Clinical Decreases
PO4= Phosphate	1.4-2.7 mEq/L SI 0.9-1.5 mmol/L	Major intracellular anion	Renal insufficiency	Diabetic ketoacidosis
Ca++ Calcium	4.5-5.8 mEq/L SI 2.1-2.6mmol/L	Essential anion for bones, teeth, mucoproteins. Role in cell membrane, muscle contraction and coagulation	Acidosis, adrenal insufficiency, diuretics (thiazide), immobilization, sarcoidosis, tumors.	Alkalosis, diarrhea, hypoproteinemia, renal insuf-ficiency, renal insuf. osteomalacia, steroid therapy, vitamin D deficiency.
Mg++ Magnesium	1.3-2.5 mEq/L SI 0.8-1.3 mmol/L	Intracellular cation, important in ATP function, acetylcholine release at N-M junction.	Antacid ingestion, parathyroidectomy, renal insufficiency	Chronic alcoholism, diabetic acidosis, diarrhea, NG Sx, severe renal disease

Hematology

Test	Normal Value	Clinical Significance	Clinical Increases	Clinical Decreases
Erythrocytes (RBCs)	Male 4.6-6.2 million/μL SI 4.6-6.2 10¹²/L Female 4.2-5.4 million/μL SI 4.2-5.4 10¹²/L	Number of cells available to carry O2/CO2	1° polycythemia 2° polycythemia from chronic hypoxemia, severe diarrhea and dehydration	Anemias, leukemia, hemorrhage followed by restored blood volume
Hemoglobin (Hgb)	Male 13-18 gm/dL SI 8.1-11.2 mmol/L Female 12-16 gm/dL SI 7.4-9.9 mmol/L	Grams of hemo-globin in 100 mL of whole blood	Polycythemia, CHF, COPD, dehydration, high altitudes.	Acute blood loss, anemias, ↑ fluid intake, pregnancy

Test	Normal Value	Clinical Significance	Clinical Increases	Clinical Decreases
Hematocrit (Hct)	Male 39-55% Female 36-48% SI 0.39-0.55 SI 0.36-0.48	% blood volume occupied by RBCs	COPD, dehydration; erythrocytosis, shock.	Acute blood loss, anemias, ↑ fluid intake, pregnancy
Reticulocytes	Male 0.5-2.7% of RBCs Female 0.5-4.1% of RBCs SI 0.005-0.015	A young RBC	↑ bone marrow activity, blood loss, infection, polycythemia, (Ruba vera)	↓ bone marrow activity, leukemia, severe anemia, aplastic anemia
RBC Sedimentation Rate	Male 0-15 mm/hr Female 0-20 mm/hr SI same	↑rate = progression of inflammation and destructive disease	Active syphilis, acute infection, menstruation, MI, pregnancy, shock, TB, tissue destruction	Allergies, CHF, fibrinogen deficiency (will be 0), newborns, polycythemia, sickle cell
Red Cell Distribution RDW	11.5% - 14.5%	Size (width) differences of RBCs.	Early indicator of anemia: iron-deficiency; folic acid deficiency; pernicious or sickle cell anemia	N/A

Test	Normal Value	Clinical Significance	Clinical Increase	Clinical Decreases
Leukocytes	Total: 5,000 - 10,000 / uL	Blood cells which	Leukocytosis: acute infections, post surgery, trauma.	Leukopenia: L shift (more immature), cancer therapy, overwhelmed or suppressed immune system.
Neutrophils (segs/bands)	40-75% bands should be near 0		Bacterial infection, neoplasm, epinephrine, steroids	
Lymphocytes	20-45%	T & B Cells	Chronic infection, viral infection (hepatitis, mono),TB.	CHF, HIV, renal failure,
Monocytes	2-10%			
Eosinophils	1-6%			Steroid therapy
Basophils	0-1%		Allergy/collagen (asthma)	
Platelet Count	150,000-400,000/μL SI 150-400 x 10^9/L	Blood constituent for clotting	COPD, high altitude, inflammation, malignancy, PE, TB, trauma, many drugs	Acute leukemia, anemias, bleeding, lupus, (many).
Bleeding Time	1-7 min (Ivy) SI 60-420 sec	Measure of platelet function	Aspirin, DIC, thrombocytopenia, uremia	
Thrombin Time	16-22 sec	Identifies prothrombin deficiency when BOTH PT and PTT are prolonged	Heparin contamination	
Prothrombin Time (PT)	10-14 sec	Extrinsic path: coumadin therapy	Clotting factor defect, liver disease, lupus erthymatosus	

Test	Normal Value	Clinical Significance	Clinical Increases	Clinical Decreases
Activated Partial Prothrombin Time (APPT)	25-39 sec Critical value >70 sec	Intrinsic path: heparin therapy monitor	Clotting factor defects, liver disease	

Chemistry

Test	Normal Value	Clinical Significance	Clinical Increases	Clinical Decreases
Acetoacetate (Acetone)	Negative	Indicator of Type 1 IDDM	Diabetic ketoacidosis	
Alpha 1-antitrypsin	< 200 mg/dL		Abceses, arthritis, early inflammation, pneumonia.	COPD
Anion Gap	7-16 mEq/L	$Na^+ - (Cl + HCO_3)$	Keto or lactic acidosis, salicylate or ethylene glycol poison, dehydration.	Various dilutional states
Aspartate Amino Transferase (AST,SGOT)	10-40 U/mL SI 0.08-0.32 μmol/sec/L	Enzyme present in heart, liver and muscle - released with injury.	MI, liver disease, pulmonary infarct, skeletal muscle disease (see CPK)	Pregnancy
Bicarbonate (HCO_3)	22-30 mEq/L SI 22-30 mmol/L	Major buffer of blood	Chronic respiratory acidosis, metabolic alkalosis(See ABGs)	Chronic respiratory alkalosis, metab. acidosis

Test	Normal Value	Clinical Significance	Clinical Increases	Clinical Decreases
BNP (b-type natriuretic peptide)	*Heart Failure:* 100-300 - Possible > 300 pg/mL - mild > 600 pg/mL - moderate > 900 pg/mL - severe	BNP is secreted from heart ventricles in response to Δ in Press when Ht. failure develops and worsens	Indicates heart failure Helps grade severity of failure	Decrease in patients taking drug therapy for heart failure, such as ACE inhibitors, beta blockers, and diuretics.
Creatine Kinase (CPK)	Male 38-174 U/L Female 26-140 U/L	Enzyme in heart, skeletal muscle	MI, muscle disease, severe exercise, polymyositis	
Creatine phospho-kinase MB Band (CPK-MB, CK-MB)	0% - 6%	Specific CK isoenzyme for heart muscle	Acute MI, severe angina pectoris, cardiac surgery, cardiac ischemia, myocarditis, hypokalemia, cardiac defibrillation	
Creatinine	0.6-1.5 mg/dL SI 53-133 μmol/L	By-product of muscle metabolism	Nephritis, renal insufficiency, urinary tract obstruction (Indicator of kidney function)	Debilitation
D-Dimer	0-500 ng/mL	fibrin fragments, adjunct test to rule out PE in some pts	PE, DVT, DIC, recent surgery, trauma, infection, liver disease, pregnancy, eclampsia, heart disease, and some CA	anticoagulant therapy (false negative)

Test	Normal Value	Clinical Significance	Clinical Increases	Clinical Decreases
Glucose	60-110 mg/dL (true) SI 3.5-5.5 mmol/L	Blood sugar	Diabetes mellitus, infections, stress, steroids, trauma, uremia	Adrenal insufficiency, insulin
HgbA$_{1c}$	Nondiabetic: 2-5% Diabetic control: 2.5-6% High average: 6.1-7.5% Diabetic uncontrol: > 8%	Long term (1-4 months) monitoring of glucose level in known diabetics	Diabetes (poorly controlled or uncontrol), hyperglycemia, recently diagnosed diabetes mellitus, alcohol ingestion, hemodialysis	Pregnancy, chronic blood loss, chronic renal failure, hemolytic anemia, conditions that decreases red blood cell life span
Insulin	4-24 μIU/mL SI 42-167 pmol/L	Pancreatic enzyme Regulates glucose metabolism	Acromegaly, insulinoma, obesity	Diabetes mellitus
Lactic Acid	5-20 mg/dL SI 0.5-1.6 mmol/L	By-product of an-aerobic metabolism	Hypoxia, CHF, ↑muscle activity, hemorrhage, shock	
Lactic Dehydrogenase (LDH)	Highly method dependent	Enzyme which catalyzes inter-conversion of lactic and pyruvate	5 Isoenzymes : Damaged cells: MI, muscle disease, liver disease, neoplastic disease, pulmonary infarction.	LDH1 > 2 = MI ↑LDH 1-5 = heart failure ↑LDH 2,3 = pulm. infarct ↑LDH 4,5 = kidney, liver ↑LDH 5 = liver disease

Test	Normal Value	Clinical Significance	Clinical Increases	Clinical Decreases
Protein	Total: 6-8 gm/dL SI 60-80 gm/L Albumin: 3.5-5.5 gm/dL SI 35-55 gm/L Globulin: 1.5-3 gm/dL SI 15-30 gm/dL	Blood proteins affecting colloidal pressure Defense proteins	Dehydration, shock Relative only Infections, erythematosus, liver disease, lupus	Hemorrhage, liver disease, leukemia, malnutr., nephrosis, neoplastic disease. Agammaglobulinemia, leukemia,malnutrition
Theophylline	10-20 mg/dL	Relaxes smooth muscle of bronchi and pulmonary blood vessels	Abdominal discomfort, anorexia, dysrhythmias, nausea, vomiting, nervousness, irritability, tachycardia	Smoking and phenytoin (Dilantin) shortens half-life
Troponin I (cTnI)	<0.35 ng/mL	Serum marker for cardiac disease. Elevates within 3 hrs of AMI Remains elevated for 5-9 days More specific then troponin T	Acute MI, minor myocardial damage, unstable angina pectoris	
Troponin T (cTnT)	<0.20 ng/L	Same as cTnI Remains elevated for 10-14 days	Same as cTnI	

Test	Normal Value	Clinical Significance	Clinical Increases	Clinical Decreases
Blood Urea Nitrogen (BUN)	8-25 mg/dL SI 2.9-8.9 mmol/L (Indicator of kidney function)	End product of protein metabolism.	Adrenal or renal insufficiency, CHF, dehydration, ↓renal flow, N2 metabolism, GI bleed, shock, urine obstruction.	Hepatic failure, low protein diet, nephrosis, pregnancy

Microbiology

Test	Normal Value	Clinical Significance	Clinical Increases	Clinical Decreases
AFB Smear and Culture	No organisms seen False negative? (5,000-50,000 organisms/mL = pos+) No growth on myobacterial agar x 6-8 wks incub is generally neg for MTb	+ Smear = poss active case of MTb (or one of 50 other species, incl. non-mycobateria spp.)	+ Culture indicates MTb present in culture site (i.e., lungs, stomach, kidneys, GI, blood, marrow, sterile body fluids, tissue, wound aspirate)	

Urine Tests

Test	Normal Value	Clinical Significance	Clinical Increases	Clinical Decreases
Urine Output	Male 900-1800 mL/day Female 600-1600 mL/day Average = 1200 mL/day	Urine output may change acid-base balance	Diuretics, diabetes insipidus, excessive intake	Dehydration, hypovolemia, injury, kidney dysfunction, shock
Urine pH	4.5-8.0	Reflects plasma pH and acid-base balance	> 7 = bacterial infection in tract, metabolic alkalosis, ↓K+, vegetarian diet	< 6 = metabolic acidosis, protein diet
Urine glucose	None present	If glucose present: indicates serum glucose level > 160-180 mg%	Diabetes	
Urine Ketones	1+ to 3+		Ketoacidosis, starvation, diet high in protein and low in carbohydrates	

5-11

Sputum Characteristics

Normal Sputum Characteristics

Amount	Color	Viscosity	Odor
10-100 cc/day	Clear	Thin	None

Type	Characteristics	Viral Pneumonia	Tuberculosis	Pulmonary infarct	Pulmonary edema	Pneumonia (Staphlococcal)	Pneumonia (Pseudomonas)	Pneumonia (Pneumococcal)	Pneumonia (Mycoplasma)	Pneumonia (Klebsiella)	Neoplasm	Lung cancer	Lung abcess	Emphysema	Cystic Fibrosis	Chronic Bronchitis	Bronchiectasis	Asthma
Mucoid	clear, thin, frothy	×	×		×				×			×		×		×		×
Purulent	yellor or green, thick, viscid, offen, odor pus		×			×	×	×					×				×	
Mucopurulent	both mucoid and purulent		×				×					×	×	×	×	×		×
Hemoptysis	bright red, frothy blood		×	×								×					×	
Currant Jelly	blood clots									×	×							
Rusty	mucopurulent with red tinge							×			×						×	
Prune Juice	dark brown, mucopurulent, offensive odor							×		×	×							
Blood-Streaked																		
Pink, frothy					×													

5-12

Sputum Collection	
Indications	To obtain sputum specimen for various laboratory testing
Contra-indications	Dependent on technique, may include: Mental Status, Age (Directed Cough), Excessive Oral Secretions, etc.
Procedure	• Explain procedure to pt • Before collection/induction, have pt blow nose and rinse out mouth • Best obtained early AM • Have pt drink extra fluids night before • Pt should sit upright when coughing • Have pt forcefully cough and spit specimen into collection cup • Do not touch edge/inside of cup • If clear/watery, probably saliva • If thick/colorful, likely good sample • Typical quantity: routine (2-3 cc), TB and fungus (10-15 cc) • Should go to lab within 1 hour • Ideal specimen is obtained by bypassing oral cavity, directly into specimen container.

Sputum Induction	
Indications	If unable to obtain sample in traditional methods, you may need to induce
Contraindications	(Relative) Patients with history of bronchospasm, asthma, etc.
Procedure	• Brief application of 3-7% hypertonic saline (consider Ultrasonic or high-output heated jet) • After nebulizing, following the Procedure above for Collection
Hazards	• May cause bronchospasm (may administer SABA prior to hypertonic to help prevent)

LABS

Confirm Order for Sputum Culture

Preparation/Collection
(see previous page)

Least Invasive

Consider the Risks vs. Benefits of each step, going from Least to Most Invasive.

Consider Hazards and Contraindications at each Step, as appropriate

Most Invasive

Directed Cough
(Huff Technique)

Addition of PEP Device

Nebulized Normal Saline
(0.9%),
Consider Hypertonic with Caution

Nasal Tracheal Suction

Recommend Bronchial Alveolar Lavage

Verify Good Sample
(quantity - 2-3 mL routinely, clean container, thick, colorful)

6 Pulmonary Function Tests

PFTs

CONTENTS

Typical Pulmonary Function Values*

Most PFT parameters do not have a single normal value. A normal or predicted value is an interactive function of BSA, age, height, weight, sex, race, etc. Also, there are no universally accepted criteria for determining degrees of abnormality.

Lung Volumes (BTPS)		
IC	Inspiratory Capacity	3.60 L
IRV	Inspiratory Reserve Volume	3.10 L
ERV	Expiratory Reserve Volume	1.20 L
VC	Vital Capacity	4.80 L
RV	Residual Volume	1.20 L
FRC	Functional Residual Capacity	2.40 L
V_{TG}	Thoracic Gas Volume	2.40 L
TLC	Total Lung Capacity	6.00 L
RV/VC	Residual Volume/VC	33%
RV/TLC	Residual Volume/TLC	20%
Ventilation (BTPS)		
V_T ●	Tidal Volume	0.50 L
RR ●	Respiratory Rate	12/min
$\dot{V}_E$ ●	Minute Volume	6.00 L/min
V_D	Dead Space Volume	150 mL
$\dot{V}_A$	Alveolar Ventilation	4.20 L/min
V_D/V_T	Dead Space/Tidal Volume Ratio	0.30

● Indicates Values that can be Measured with Bedside Spirometry

Mechanics of Breathing

FVC ●	Forced Vital Capacity	4.80 L
SVC ●	Slow Vital Capacity	4.80 L
FIVC	Forced Inspiratory Vital Capacity	4.80 L
FEV$_T$ ●	Forced Exp Volume over Time	(varies)
FEV 1%	Forced Exp Volume Ratio (1 sec)	83%
FEV 3%	Forced Exp Volume Ratio (3 secs)	97%
FEF ● 200-1200	Forced Expiratory Flow from 200cc to 1200cc	400 L/min
PEF ●	Peak Expiratory Flow	600 L/min
FEF 25-75 ●	Forced Expiratory Flow from 25-75% of FVC	4.70 L/sec
FIF 25-75 (FIFmax)	Forced Inspiratory Flow from 25-75% of FIVC	5.00 L/sec
$\dot{V}$max 50	Forced Expiratory Flow at 50% of FVC	5.00 L/sec
MVV ●	Maximal Voluntary Ventilation	170 L/min
C$_L$	Static Compliance of Lungs	0.2 L/cm H$_2$O
C$_{LT}$	Static Compliance of Lungs and Thoracic Cage	0.1 L/cm H$_2$O
Raw	Airway Resistance	1.50 cmH2O/L/sec
Rpul	Pulmonary Resistance	2.00 cmH2O/L/sec
Gaw	Airway Conductance	0.66 L/sec/cmH$_2$O
SGaw	Specific Conductance	0.22 L/sec/cmH$_2$O/L
W rest	Work of Quiet Breathing	0.5 kg • M/min
W max	Maximal Work of Breathing	10 kg • M/breath
MIP ●	Maximal Inspiratory Pressure	- 80 mm Hg
MEP	Maximal Expiratory Pressure	120 mm Hg

Distribution of Inspired Gas

$\dot{V}$A	Alveolar Ventilation	4.20 L/min
V$_D$/V$_T$	Physiological Deadspace Ratio	< 30
SBN$_2$	Single-Breath N$_2$ Test ΔN$_2$ from 750-1250 mL expired	< 1.5% N$_2$
7 Minute N$_2$	Alveolar N$_2$ after 7 min of O$_2$	< 2.5% N$_2$
CV	Closing Volume	400 mL
CV/VC	Closing Volume/VC Ratio	9%
CC	Closing Capacity	1600 mL
CC/TLC	Closing Capacity/TLC Ratio	32%
Slope of Phase III in Single-Breath N$_2$ Test		< 2% N$_2$/L

● Indicates Values that can be Measured with Bedside Spirometry

Pulmonary Blood Flow		
CO	Cardiac Output	5.40 L/min
$\dot{Q}T$	Total Perfusion of the Lung	5.20 L/min
$\dot{Q}Sphys$	Physiological shunt	< 7%
$\dot{Q}Sanat$	Anatomic shunt	< 3%
QCpul	Pulmonary Cap. Blood Volume	75-100 mL

Alveolar Ventilation/Perfusion		
$\dot{V}A$	Alveolar Ventilation	4.20 L/min
$\dot{Q}Cpul$	Pulmonary Capillary Blood Flow	5.20 L/min
$\dot{V}A/\dot{Q}C$	Alveolar Ventilation/Blood Flow	0.8

Gas Exchange		
$\dot{V}CO_2$	CO_2 Production	200 mL/min
$\dot{V}O_2$	O_2 Consumption	250 mL/min
RQ	Respiratory Quotient ($\dot{V}CO_2/\dot{V}O_2$)	0.8 (tissue level)
RER	Respiratory Exchange Ratio (CO_2 output / O_2 uptake)	0.8 (end-tidal level)

Alveolar Gas		
PAO_2	Partial Press of Alveolar O_2	109 mm Hg
$PACO_2$	Partial Press of Alveolar CO_2	40 mm Hg

Arterial Blood		
PaO_2	Partial Press of Arterial PaO_2	99 mm Hg
SaO_2	O_2 Saturation of Arterial Blood	97%
pH	Negative log of H^+ concentration	7.40
$PaCO_2$	Partial Press of Arterial CO_2	40 mm Hg
PaO_2 on 100	P.P. While Breathing 100% O_2	640 mm Hg
$PA-aO_2$	A-aO_2 Gradient	10 mm Hg
$PA-aO_2$	A-aO_2 Gradient on 100% O_2	33 mm Hg
CaO_2	Content of Arterial O_2	20 vol%
$C\bar{V}O_2$	Content of Mixed Venous O_2	15 vol%
$Ca-\bar{V}O_2$	A-V difference of O_2 Content	5 vol%

Diffusion		
$DLCO$	Diffusing Capacity (Single Breath)	25/17mL/min/ mmHg
$DL/\dot{V}A$	Diffusing Capacity/$\dot{V}A$ (KCO)	4

Control Of Ventilation	
Ventilatory Response to Hypercapnia	0.50 L/min/mmHg
Ventilatory Response to Hypoxia	0.20 L/min/ΔSO_2
Arterial Blood PO_2 during Moderate Excerise	95 mm Hg

* Typical values for a young male at sea level.
  Height 165 cm, weight 64 kg, body surface area 1.7 m^2.

Overview Of Patterns Of Abnormal Pulmonary Functions

PF Tests	Obstructive				
	Asthma	Emphysema	Chronic Bronchitis	Small Airways Disease	
Lung Volumes					
SVC	N↓	N↓	N↓	N	↓
RV	↑	↑	↑	N↑	N↓
FRC	↑	↑	↑	N	N↓
TLC	N↑	↑	N↑	N	↓
RV/TLC	↑	↑	↑	N↑	N↑
Mechanics					
FVC	↓	↓	N↓	N	↓
FEV1	↓	↓	↓	N	N
FEF 200-1200	N↓	N↓	↓	N	N↓
FEF 25-75	↓	↓	↓	↓	N↓
PEF	↓	↓	↓	N	N↓
MVV	↓	↓	↓	N	N↓
Cstat	N	↑	N	N	↓
Cdyn	↓	↓	↓	N↓	↓
Raw	↑	N↓	↑	N	N
CV	↑	↑	↑	N↑	N↑
V/Q Relationships					
A-a Gradient	↑	↑	↑	↑	N↑
$\dot{Q}s/\dot{Q}_T$	↑	↑	↑	↑	N↑
V_D/V_T	↑	↑	↑	N↑	↑
D_LCO	N	↓	N	N	N↓

N = Normal, ↑ = Increased, ↓ = Decreased

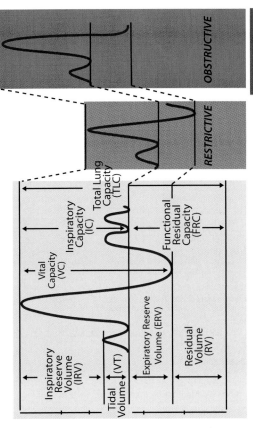

OBSTRUCTIVE

RESTRICTIVE

Total Lung Capacity (TLC)

Inspiratory Capacity (IC)

Functional Residual Capacity (FRC)

Vital Capacity (VC)

Inspiratory Reserve Volume (IRV)

Tidal Volume (VT)

Expiratory Reserve Volume (ERV)

Residual Volume (RV)

Volumes and Capacities
(see 6-1 for values)
(see 6-7 for descriptions of maneuvers)

Guidelines for Severity of Lung Volume Disorders

General Guidelines for Assignment of Severity of Lung Volume Disorders

Volume (Normal)	Disorder	Severity		
		Mild	Moderate	Severe
TLC (80-120% Pred)	Restrictive	70-80%	60-70%	< 60%
	Obstructive	120-130%	130-150%	> 150%
VC (> 90% Pred)	Restrictive	70-90%	50-70%	< 50%
	Obstructive	70-90%	50-70%	< 50%
FRC (65-135% Pred)	Restrictive	55-65%	45-55%	< 45%
	Obstructive	135-150%	150-200%	> 200%
RV (65-135% Pred)	Restrictive	55-65%	45-55%	< 45%
	Obstructive	135-150%	150-250%	>250%

Adapted from Madama, V., *Pulmonary Function Testing and Cardiopulmonary Stress Testing*. Copyright 1993 by Delmar Publishers.

Restriction
- Most all values are ↓ proportionately (esp. VC, TLC).
- Normal flows

Obstruction
- ↑TLC, ↑RV, ↑FRC, ↑RV/VC, ↑RV/TLC, ↓ VC, & ↓ Flows

Pulmonary Function Tests

Spirometry
Lung Volumes and Capacities

Test	Description
Tidal Volume (V$_T$)	Volume of gas moved in or out of the lungs in a normal resting breath.
Inspiratory Reserve Volume (IRV)	Maximum volume of gas inspired from end-tidal inspiration.
Inspiratory Capacity (IC)	Maximum volume of gas inspired from resting expiratory level (VT + IRV).
Expiratory Reserve Volume (ERV)	Maximum volume of gas expired from resting expiratory level.
Vital Capacity (VC)	Maximum volume of gas expired after a maximum inspiration (IC + ERV).
Residual Volume (RV)	Volume of gas in the lungs at the end of a maximum expiration.
Total Lung Capacity (TLC)	Volume of gas in lungs at the end of a maximum inspiration.
RV/TLC	Residual volume expressed as a percent of total lung capacity.
Functional Residual Capacity (FRC)	Volume in lungs at resting expiratory level (ERV + RV).
Thoracic Gas Volume (V$_{TG}$)	Volume of gas in entire thoracic cavity at resting expiratory level whether or not it communicates with the airways.

Normal Values
- Normal values may vary within 20% of predicted.
- Values will change with position, age, sex, height, altitude, race/ethnicity.

Other Tests for Measuring Lung Volumes
- Helium (He) Dilution: Measures RV + FRC
- Nitrogen (N$_2$) Washout: Measures RV + FRC
- Body Plethysmography: Measures V$_{TG}$ (FRC) + Raw

Pulmonary Mechanics

Test		Interpretation
Slow Vital Capacity (SVC)	Maximum volume of gas exhaled slowly after a maximum inspiration.	Both SVC and FVC are effort dependent. SVC should = FVC.
Forced Vital Capacity (FVC)	Maximum volume of gas exhaled forcefully after a maximum inspiration.	Restrictive: ↓SVC & ↓FVC; Obstructive: SVC may be normal, ↓FVC > ↓SVC
Forced Expiratory Volume, timed (FEVt)	A volume of gas measured at a specific time interval during an FVC maneuver.	
Forced Expiratory Volume, percent (FEVt%, FEVt/FVC)	The percent of gas forcefully exhaled during an FVC maneuver.	<table> Time | % | Normal | Obstructive | Restrictive; 0.5 | 60; 1.0 | 83 | >70% | <70% | >70% usually; 2.0 | 94 </table>
Forced Expiratory Flow 25-75% (FEF25-75, MMEF, MMF)	Average forced expiratory flow during the middle half of an FVC (mid-maximal expiratory flow).	Measures average flow through small airways. Normal = 4.7 L/sec (282 L/min). ↓ in early stages of obstructive. Normal in restrictive.
Forced Expiratory Flow 200-1200 (FEF200-1200, MEF)	Average forced expiratory flow of one liter of gas after the first 200 mL is exhaled during an FVC (maximal expiratory flow).	Measures average flow through larger airways. Normal = 6-7 L/sec (400 L/min). ↓ = mechanical problem or severe obstruction. Effort dependent.
Peak Expiratory Flow (PEF, FEFmax)	Maximum instantaneous flow attained during an FVC maneuver.	Indication of ability to cough. Normal = 10 L/sec (600 L/min).

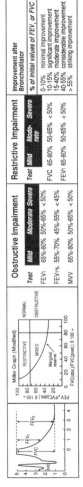

Peak Inspiratory Flow (PIF)	Maximum instantaneous flow attained during a forceful inspiration.	Helpful in distinguishing between obstruction vs. lack of effort (Very effort dependent). Normal = 5 L/sec (300 L/min). PIF > PEF in obstruction, PIF = PEF in restriction.
Maximum Voluntary Ventilation (MVV, MBC)	Total volume of gas a subject can breathe in and out with maximum effort in one minute (maximum breathing capacity).	Indicates efficiency of total pulmonary system: muscles, compliance, resistance, neurological coordination. Very effort dependent. ↓ with moderate obstruction (exaggerates air-trapping) and severe restriction.

Obstructive Impairment

Test	Mild	Moderate	Severe
FEV1	65%-80%	50%-65%	<50%
FEV1%	55%-70%	45%-55%	<45%
MVV	65%-80%	50%-65%	<50%

Restrictive Impairment

Test	Mild	Moderate	Severe
FVC	65-80%	50-65%	<50%
FEV1	65-80%	50-65%	<50%

Improvement after Bronchodilator

% of initial values of FEV1 or FVC	
0-10%	minimal improvement
10-15%	significant improvement
15-40%	moderate improvement
40-55%	considerable improvement
> 55%	striking improvement

6-9

Compliance and Resistance

Test		Interpretation
Static Compliance (Cstat)	A measure of the distensibility of the lungs and thorax (i.e., pressure required to maintain a given volume of inflation).	Normal: 0.1 L/cm H₂O. Represents elasticity of lungs and recoil of thorax. ↓Cstat = ↑ elastic recoil, ↑Cstat = ↓ elastic recoil See Ch 7 and Equations, Ch 9.
Dynamic Compliance (Cdyn)	A measure of the distensibility of the lungs and thorax during breathing (i.e., pressure required to obtain a given volume of inflation).	Represents a combination of Cstat and Raw. See Ch 7 and Equations, Ch 9.
Frequency Dependent Compliance	Cdyn measured at rapid breathing rates.	Normal > 80%. Sensitive indicator of small airway disease (↑ rate → ↓compliance).
Airway Resistance (Raw)	Ratio of alveolar pressure to airflow. See Ch 7 and Equations, Ch 9.	Measurement of the flow-resistive properties of the airways. Norm= 0.6-2.4 cm H₂O/L/sec @ flow of 0.5 L/sec². Varies inversely with lung vol.

Test	Description	Interpretation
Flow Volume Loop (Curve) (MEF + MIF) Adapted from Madama, V. Pulmonary Function Testing and Cardiopulmonary Stress Testing. Copyright 1993 by Delmar publishers.	Test of flow and volume relationships during maximal inspiratory and expiratory maneuvers. $\dot{V}$max 75 = max flow at 75 % of FVC (50 = 50%, 25 = 25%)	Test of small airway disease. Shapes of curves are qualitative diagnostic tests. Flow at lower 2/3 volume becomes less effort-dependent. $\dot{V}$max provides a quantitative value of flow.
$\Delta\dot{V}$max 50	Difference in $\Delta\dot{V}$50 when using two gases of differing densities.	Less dense gas = ↓ resistance at ↑ lung volumes, where airflow is turbulent. Laminar flow predominates at lower lung volumes where resistance is independent of gas density. The lung volume at which the gas density begins to effect is called the **Viso** $\dot{V}$. Small airway disease with↑resistance causes site of flow limitation to occur at ↑ volumes.
Viso $\dot{V}$	Volume of lungs at which flows become identical using two gases of different density (i.e., flow independent of density)	

6-11

Gas Distribution

Test	Interpretation
Single Breath Nitrogen Washout (SBN₂) or Single Breath O₂ Test (SBO₂) (ΔN₂ 750-1250)	Rise in N_2 in 500 mL of exhaled gas after exhalation of the first 750 mL following inhalation of 100% O_2.	Index of evenness of ventilation. Normal (even) ventilation = rise of N_2 % along Phase 3 < 1.5%. > 1.5% = uneven distribution and/or uneven expiratory flow. (See next pg)
Closing Volume (CV)	Volume of gas expired between onset of airway closure (Phase 4) and RV. Expressed as % of FVC. Normal < 10%. ↑CV = early obstruction, age, CHF, restriction when FRC < CV. Sensitive test to measure point of small airway closure. Used to determine evenness of ventilation. Basilar airways close first ($\downarrow O_2$). Remainder of exhaled air is from apical airways ($\uparrow N_2$).
Closing Capacity (CC)	Closing volume plus RV. Expressed as % of TLC.	CC = measurement of choice because it includes the ↑RV in obstructive disorders. Normal < 32%. ↑ CV/VC and CC/TLC = obstructive
Nitrogen Washout Test (7 minute)	Concentration of N_2 remaining in alveolar gas after 7 minutes of breathing 100% O_2.	Washout curve is indicative of distribution of ventilation. Normal = < 2.5% (See next pg)
Radioxenon Lung Scan (133Xe)	Radiographic scan of lung using radioisotope 133 Xe	Determines how rapidly and how even the gas is distributed. Washing out shows areas of ↑ ventilation and/or trapped gas.

Nitrogen Washout Test

Single Breath Nitrogen Washout Test (SBN2)

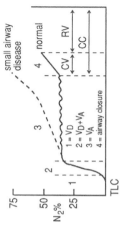

Dead Space Ratio (V_D/V_T)	Ratio of volume of gas not participating in gas exchange in a normal breath compared to total volume of the breath.	Normal < 0.3 (1 mL/lb IBW). Estimate of functional lung capacity and indication of V/Q equality. ↑ ratio = ↑ V_D = ↑ wasted ventilation. See Ch 9
Alveolar Ventilation ($\dot{V}_A$)	Volume of gas/unit time (L/min) participating in gas exchange.	Normal = 4-5 L/min with wide variation. Calculation less accurate as V/Q inequality increases. See Ch 9

Blood Flow Distribution

Test		Interpretation
Single Breath CO_2 Elimination	Measurement of CO_2 concentration during exhalation. % CO_2 vs time graph: abnormal, normal curves 1 = VD 2 = VD+VA 3 = VA	Index of uniformity of ventilation to blood flow. Uneven V/Q → different CO_2 in different lung areas and different emptying rates → linear curve.
Clinical Shunt (Qs/Qt)	Quantitative measurement of fraction of blood passing by the lungs and not participating in gas exchange.	Normal = 3-5%. ↑shunt = ↑ V/Q = ↑ amount of mixed venous blood not coming in contact with alveolar air. See Equations, Ch 9.
Radioxenon Elimination (133Xe)	Qualitative view of Xe diffusing from the blood into the lungs.	Analysis of V/Q equality.
Angiogram	Roetgenogram view of the pulmonary vessels	Qualitative analysis of lung perfusion.
Lung Perfusion Scan	Photoscintography of lung perfusion	

Diffusion Capacity

| Single Breath or Steady State (D$_L$CO$_{SB}$ or SS) | Tests to measure all factors affecting diffusion across A-C membrane.

Normal = 25 mL CO/min/mm Hg. | D$_L$CO is also directly related to alveolar volume.
Normal D$_L$CO/$\dot{V}A$ = 4 (20 mL/min/mm Hg/5L).
↓ D$_L$CO (due to ↓ $\dot{V}A$) = restriction
↓ D$_L$CO (due to V/Q mismatch; uneven inspired volume/alveolar volume) = obstruction. |

Reference equations vary widely, particularly for DLCO where often cited values are based upon people who have never smoked with various age-ranges. *

It is advisable, therefore, to review PFT results in context of the patient's quality-of-life.

* from Miller & Enright. PFT Interpretive Strategies: American Thoracic Society/ European Respiratory Society 2005 Guideline Gaps. Respiratory Care, Volume 57, Issue 1, 2012.

Simplified Algorithm for Assessing Lung Function*

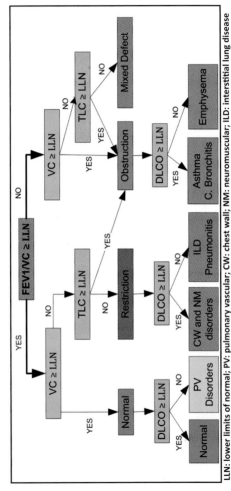

LLN: lower limits of normal; PV: pulmonary vascular; CW: chest wall; NM: neuromuscular; ILD: interstitial lung disease

Reprinted with permission[1]. See notes and explanations on the next page.

*Note:
Two LLNs are currently in use.

1. LLN % - Many PFT labs still use LLN%
(i.e., 80% of the predicted value for FEV1and FVC; and 70% of the predicted value for FEV1/FVC ratio). The use of a fixed percentage completely ignores changes in predicted values due to age, height, sex, and race/ethnic group, and can lead to important errors in interpreting lung function, and is therefore, no longer recommended.

The ATS/ERS Statement on COPD and GOLD COPD Standards defines COPD as a post-bronchodilator FEV1/FVC ratio < 0.7. This is an oversimplification and approximation meant for initial screening purposes only, and is not meant to be applied in the PFT lab as the true LLN for all populations.

2. LLN CI - In the USA, the more valid and currently recommended approach by the ATS/ERS Pulmonary Function Testing Guidelines, is to define the LLN as the lower fifth percentile, or 95% confidence limit, of the predicted value (LLN CI), (i.e., the value exceeded by 95% of normal individuals of the same gender, age, height, and race/ethnic group).

ATS/ERS also recommends adoption of the NHANES III (National Health and Nutrition Examination Survey) reference equations for adults, for predicted normals.

---

1. ATS/ERS Task Force: Standardization of Lung Function Testing, Series #5; Pellegrino, R., et al., Interpretative strategies for lung function tests. The European Respiratory Journal , 26 (5), 948-968, 2005.

2. Aggarwal, A., et al., Comparison of fixed percentage method and lower confidence limits for defining limits of normality for interpretation of spirometry. Respiratory Care , Vol 51, #7, 2006.

Mechanics of Ventilation

Volume & Pressure Changes During Spont. Breathing

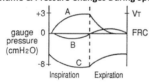

Inspiration	Diaphragm/chest muscles contract → ↑intrathoracic vol. → ↓ intrathoracic (pleural) pressure + pleural cohesion → ↑ intrapulmonary (lung) vol → ↓ intrapulmonary (alveoli) pressure → air moves down gradient (in).
Active	
Expiration	Muscles relax, plus elastic recoil of lung → ↓ intrapulmonary vol- ume → ↑intrapulmonary press → air moves down gradient (out).
Passive	

Pressures and Pressure Gradients

A: Lung Volume
B: Alveolar Pressure
C: Intrathoracic Pressure

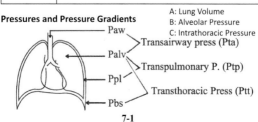

Pressures*

Abbreviation	Definition	Also Known As	
Paw, Pawo, or Pm	Pressure at airway (opening or mouth)	Mouth pressure	Normally atmospheric (zero), unless positive airway pressure is applied
Palv	Pressure in the alveoli	Intrapulmonary pressure, alveoli pressure (P_A)	Varies during breathing cycle
Ppl	Pressure in pleural space	Intrapleural pressure (P_{pl}) or intrathoracic pressure (P_{IT})	Varies during breathing cycle. Normally negative during quiet spontaneous breathing
Patm or Pbs	Pressure at body surface	Atmospheric (barometric) pressure (P_B)	Normally zero, unless negative pressure is applied

Pressure Gradients

Pta	Transairway pressure gradient, Pta = Paw - Palv	Pressure difference down the airway.	Responsible for gas flow into and out of the lungs.
Ptp	Transpulmonary pressure gradient, Ptp = Palv - Ppl	Pressure difference across the lung.	Responsible for degree of and maintenance of alveolar inflation or volume change.
Ptt	Transthoracic pressure gradient, Ptt = Patm - Palv	Pressure difference across the lung and chest wall.	Total pressure necessary to expand or contract the lungs and chest wall together.

Clinical Note: Transrespiratory pressure gradient = Paw – Pbs.

Transmural pressure gradient (Ptm) = Pressure gradient across a vessel wall (intravascular pressure [P_{IV}] minus P_{IT}).

* Pressures are measured as gauge pressure in cm H_2O and expressed relative to atmospheric pressure. Hence, a pressure of 5 cm H_2O is atmospheric (1034 cm H_2O) plus 5 cm H_2O.

Compliance

(See Chapter 9 for clinical equations)

Compliance = ease of distention
= 1/difficulty of distention (static impedance)
= 1/elastance
= 1/elastic forces + surface tension

↑ Elastance = ↓ Compliance	↓ Elastance = ↑Compliance

Static Compliance (Cstat)	Total compliance of lung and thorax $C_{LT} = \Delta V/\Delta P$	
Dynamic Compliance (Cdyn)	Total impendance $Cdyn = Cstat = Raw$	
Airway Resistance (Raw)	Impedance to Airflow $Raw = \Delta P/flow$ = 0.6 - 2.4 cmH$_2$O/L/sec @ 0.5 L/sec (norm)	
Time Constant (TC)	Filling or Emptying Time of the Lung (Cstat x Raw) - See Chapter 9	
Time Constant Examples	**Normal Lung Unit**	TC = 0.1 L/cmH$_2$O x 2.0 cmH$_2$O/L/Sec = (0.1) x (4.0) = 0.2 sec
	Asthma	TC = 0.1 L/cmH$_2$O x 4.0 cmH$_2$O/L/Sec = (0.1) x (2.0) = 0.4 sec
	Fibrosis	TC = 0.05 L/cmH$_2$O x 2.0 H$_2$O/L/Sec = (0.05) x (2.0) = 0.1 sec

SEE FIGURE NEXT PAGE

A **Long Time Constant** results in alveoli that fill slowly on inspiration (so take even longer to empty)

A **Short Time Constant** results in alveoli that fill and empty quickly

Expiratory Airway Resistance is usually higher than Inspiratory Resistance.

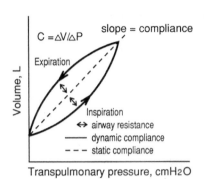

Distribution of Ventilation

Minute Ventilation ($\dot{V}_E$)	Total air moved in or out of the lungs in one minute ($V_T \times f$) ($\dot{V}_A + \dot{V}_D$)
Alveolar Ventilation ($\dot{V}_A$)	Ventilation which participates in gas exchange ($V_A \times f$) ($\dot{V}_E - \dot{V}_D$)
Deadspace Ventilation ($\dot{V}_D$)	Ventilation which does not participate in gas exchange ($V_D \times f$) ($\dot{V}_E - \dot{V}_A$)

Types of Deadspace

VDphys	=	VDanat	+	VDalv	+	VDmech
Physiological (Total)	=	*Anatomical* Conducting passages, 1/3 V_T or 1cc/lb IBW, ↓ ½ with trach	+	Alveolar Alveoli without perfusion	+	Mechanical Air in tubing that is rebreathed.

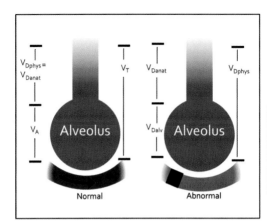

Normal / Abnormal

Distribution of Ventilation through Lung Regions

Spontaneous Ventilation: Air moving into the lungs at FRC will go to the gravity-dependent areas. Near TLC distribution will be more even.

Mechanical Ventilation (Positive Pressure): Air will take the path of least resistance, usually the uppermost areas. This is why large tidal volumes (10-15 mL/kg PBW) *were* sometimes given - so that air will fill the uppermost portions and then move into the gravity dependent portions where most of the perfusion is.

While large tidal volumes may distribute physiologically, it is important to remember that lung units are often not "homogenous" (one single unit). Because of this, current evidence-based medicine supports delivered tidal volumes in the 6-8 mL/kg PBW range (or less). The goal is to protect healthy lung units which are often more compliant - air will follow the path of least resistance.

Perfusion

$\dot{Q}_T$ = Total perfusion of the lung ($\approx$ CO) = ($\dot{Q}_c + \dot{Q}_s$)
$\dot{Q}_c$ = Capillary perfusion (blood participating in gas exchange)
$\dot{Q}_s$ = Shunt (blood not participating in gas exchange)

$\dot{Q}_{sphys}$ =	$\dot{Q}_{sanat}$ +	$\dot{Q}_{scap}$
Physiological Shunt (Total)	Anatomical Shunt Universal = 2 - 5% CO. Pleural, thebesian, & bronchial veins, congenital heart defects, AV malformations, vascular lung tumors.	Capillary Shunt Alveolar collapse, pneumothorax, airway obstruction, ↓surfactant, atelectasis, space occupying lesions, alveolar filling (secretions, edema, abscess, pneumonia), diffusion defect.

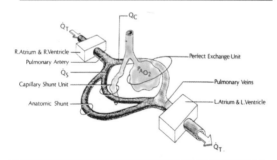

Perfusion Zones

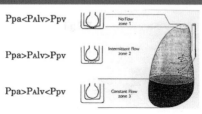

Zone levels are dependent on cardiac output, alveolar pressure (vol, esp. PEEP), and gravity. Most blood flow occurs in zone 3, which will be the gravity dependent areas.

Body position has a significant effect on the distribution of pulmonary blood flow, as shown in the erect (A), supine (lying on the back) (B), and lateral (lying on the side) (C), positions.

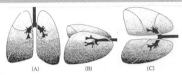

(A)   (B)   (C)

Above figures reprinted with permission from Shapiro, B, et.al.: Clinical Application of Arterial Blood Gases, 3rd Ed., Yearbook Publishers, 1982.

Ventilation/Perfusion ($\dot{V}/\dot{Q}$)

Normal Lung = $\dot{V}/\dot{Q}$ = 4 L/min / 5 L/min = 0.8 (normal ratio)

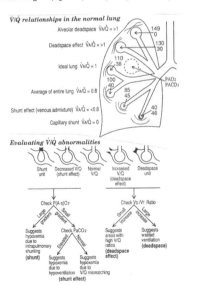

Adapted from Harper, R.W.: A Guide to Respiratory Care: Phys. & Clin. Applic. Copyright 1981 by J.B. Lippincott Co., Philadelphia.

8 Cardiovascular Dynamics

Hemodynamic Parameters

Measured		Abbreviation	Normal Value
Arterial Blood Pressure	Systolic	BPsys	100-140 mmHg
	Mean	$\overline{BP}$ or MAP	70-105 mmHg
	Diastolic	BPdia	60-80 mmHg
	Pulse Pressure	PP	20-80 mmHg
Cardiac Output		CO	4-8 L/min
Central Venous Pressure		CVP	0-6 mmHg / 0-8 cmH₂O
Heart Rate		HR	60-100 beats/min
Pulmonary Artery Pressures (PAP)	Systolic	PASP	15-25 mmHg
	Mean	PAMP or $\overline{PAP}$	10-15 mmHg
	Diastolic	PADP	8-15 mmHg
	End Diastolic	PAEDP	0-12 mmHg
	Wedge	PAWP	4-12 mmHg
Right Atrial Pressure		RAP or $\overline{RAP}$	0-6 mmHg
Right Ventricular End Diastolic Pressure		RVEDP	0-5 mmHg
Right Ventricular End Systolic Pressure		RVESP	15-25 mmHg

Derived	Abbrev.	Normal Value
Body Surface Area	BSA	See chapter 9
Cardiac Index	CI	2.5-4.4 L/min/m^2
Left Atrial Pressure	LAP	4-12 mmHg
Left Ventricular End Diastolic Pressure	LVEDP	4-12 mmHg
Left Ventricular End Systolic Pressure	LVESP	100-140 mmHg
Left Ventricular Stroke Work	LVSW	60-80 gm/m/beat
Left Ventricular Stroke Work Index	LVSWI	40-75 gm/m/beat/m^2
Pulmonary Vascular Resistance	PVR	20-200 dynes•sec•cm^{-5} 0.25-2.5 units (mmHg/L/min)
Pulmonary Vascular Resistance Index	PVRI	30-350 dynes•sec•cm^{-5}/m^2
Right Ventricular Stroke Work	RVSW	10-15 gm/m/beat
Right Ventricular Stroke Work Index	RVSWI	4-12 gm/m/beat/m^2
Stroke Volume	SV	60-120 mL/beat
Stroke Volume Index	SVI	35-75 mL/beat/m^2
Systemic Vascular Resistance	SVR	800-1600 dynes•sec•cm^{-5} 10-20 units (mmHg/L/min)
Systemic Vascular Resistance Index	SVRI	1400-2600 dynes•sec•cm^{-5}/m^2

Other Hemodynamic Parameters

Non-Invasive	Invasive			
Measured	Measured		Derived	
Capillary Refill	$PaCO_2$	PvO_2	$PA\text{-}aO_2$	$\dot{D}O_2$
$PtcCO_2$	PaO_2	$P\bar{v}O_2$	$Pa\text{-}vO_2$	LV Fx Curve
$PtcO_2$	pH	SaO_2	$Pa\text{-}\bar{v}O_2$	$M\dot{D}O_2$
SaO_2 (SpO_2)	$PvCO_2$	SvO_2	CaO_2	$M\dot{V}O_2$
Skin color/dryness	$P\bar{v}CO_2$	$S\bar{v}O_2$	$Ca\text{-}\bar{v}O_2$	O_2ER
Temp (core/skin)			CvO_2	$\dot{Q}S/\dot{Q}T$
UO			$C\bar{v}O_2$	$\dot{V}O_2$

See Chapter 9 for equations and their significance.

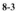

Cardiopulmonary

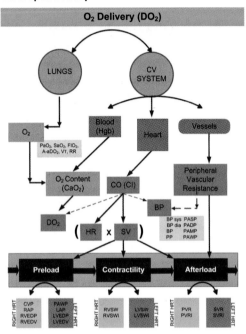

Reprinted with permission from Oakes, D.; *Hemodynamic Monitoring: A Bedside Reference Manual*. Copyright 2017 by Health Educator Publications, Inc.

OVERVIEW OF O2 DELIVERY EQUATIONS

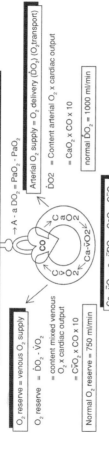

$\rightarrow$ A - a $DO_2 = PaO_2 - PaO_2$

Arterial O_2 supply = O_2 delivery ($\dot{D}O_2$) (O_2↑transport)

$\dot{D}O2$ = Content arterial O_2 x cardiac output

= CaO_2 x CO x 10

normal $\dot{D}O_2$ = 1000 ml/min

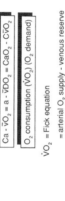

O_2 extraction ratio (O_2 ER) =
$\dfrac{O_2 \text{ consumption (demand)}}{O_2 \text{ delivery (supply)}}$

$O_2 ER = \dfrac{\dot{V}O_2}{\dot{D}O_2}$ x 100

Normal O_2ER = 25%

O_2 reserve = venous O_2 supply

O_2 reserve = $\dot{D}O_2 - \dot{V}O_2$

= content mixed venous O_2 x cardiac output

= $C\bar{v}O_2$ x CO x 10

Normal O_2 reserve = 750 ml/min

Ca - $\bar{v}O_2$ = a - $\bar{v}DO_2$ = $CaO_2 - C\bar{v}O_2$

O_2 consumption ($\dot{V}O_2$) (O_2 demand)

$\dot{V}O_2$ = Fick equation

= arterial O_2 supply - venous reserve

= (CaO_2 x CO) - ($C\bar{v}O_2$ x CO) x 10

= Ca - $\bar{v}O_2$ x CO x 10

normal $\dot{V}O_2$ = 250 ml/min

Reprinted with permission from Oakes, D; Hemodynamic Monitoring: A Bedside Reference Manual. Copyright 1995 by Health Educator Publications, Inc.

Blood Flow through the Heart

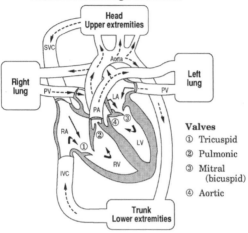

Valves

① Tricuspid
② Pulmonic
③ Mitral (bicuspid)
④ Aortic

Factors Controlling Blood Pressure

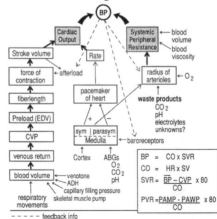

$$BP = CO \times SVR$$

$$CO = HR \times SV$$

$$SVR = \frac{\overline{BP} - CVP}{CO} \times 80$$

$$PVR = \frac{PAMP - PAWP}{CO} \times 80$$

- - - - feedback info

8-6

Overview of Cardiopulmonary Pressure Dynamics

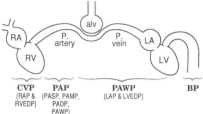

CVP	PAP	PAWP	BP
(RAP & RVEDP)	(PASP, PAMP, PADP, PAWP)	(LAP & LVEDP)	

A-Line Monitoring

Arterial Pressures

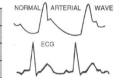

BPsys	120 mmHg
BPdia	80 mmHg
$\overline{BP}$ (MAP)	93 mmHg
PP	40 mmHg

(see page 8-1 for normal ranges)
(See page 8-9 to 8-10 for some disease-causing variations)

Arterial Waveform

CVP Monitoring

Venous Pressure

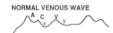

CVP	0-6 mmHg
	0-8 cmH$_2$O

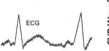

(See page 8-9 to 8-10 for some disease-causing variations)

CVP Waveform

See Oakes' Hemodynamic Monitoring:
A Bedside Reference Manual
• Indications, Insertion Sites, Equipment, Techniques, Maintenance, Infection Control, Samples, Pressure and Waveform Variations, Complications, Troubleshooting, and removal of Lines

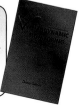

PAP MONITORING[1]

Measurements Obtainable:

Measured	Derived	
CO	CI	Note: All invasive parameters may be obtained with the combination of an A-Line and a PA line (thermodiulution)
CVP	CvO_2	
HR	$C\bar{v}O_2$	
PADP	LV (function,	
PASP	curve)	**A-Line**
PAWP (LAP,	LVSW	**+**
LVEDP)	LVSWI	**PA Line parameters**
pHv	PAMP	**Derived**
pH$\bar{v}$	PVR	
$PvCO_2$	PVRI	$a-vDO_2$ $\quad$ $\dot{M}DO_2$
$P\bar{v}CO_2$	RVSW	$a-\bar{v}DO_2$ $\quad$ $\dot{M}\bar{V}O_2$
PvO_2	RVSWI	$Ca-vO_2$ $\quad$ O_2ER
$P\bar{v}O_2$	SV	$Ca-\bar{v}O_2$ $\quad$ $\dot{Q}_s/\dot{Q}_T$
RAP (RVEDP)	SVI	CPP $\quad$ SVR
SvO_2	SW	$\dot{D}O_2$ $\quad$ SVRI
$S\bar{v}O_2$	SWI	VO_2

Pressures		Waveforms
CVP	0-6 mmHg	
RVSP	15-25 mmHg	
RVEDP	0-6 mmHg	
PASP	15-25 mmHg	
PADP	8-15 mmHg	
PAMP	10-15 mmHg	
PAWP	4-12 mmHg	
PADP-PAWP gradient	0-6 mmHg	

* All pressures should be measured at end-expiration (see page 8-9 and 8-10 for some disease-causing variations.

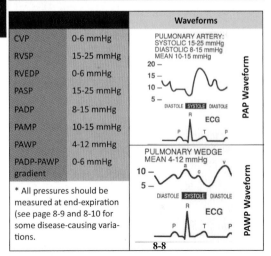

PULMONARY ARTERY:
SYSTOLIC 15-25 mmHg
DIASTOLIC 8-15 mmHg
MEAN 10-15 mmHg

DIASTOLE SYSTOLE DIASTOLE

ECG

PAP Waveform

PULMONARY WEDGE
MEAN 4-12 mmHg

DIASTOLE SYSTOLE DIASTOLE

ECG

PAWP Waveform

8-8

Some Disease Entities Causing PRESSURE Changes

BP	CVP		PAP	PCWP
Increased Aortic Insufficiency Arteriosclerosis Drugs (inotropes, vasopressors) Essential Hypertension	**Increased** ↑Preload: Hypervolemia Tricuspid Insufficiency VSD ↑Afterload: ARDS COPD Chronic LVF Cor Pulmonale Hypoxemia MV esp. with PEEP Pulmonic Stenosis PVR↑ (emboli, hypertension) Tricuspid Stenosis	**↓ Contractility:** Cardiac Tamponade Cardiomyopathy Constrictive Pericarditis LVF (CHF, MI, shock) MI (esp. RH) RVF	**Increased** Cardiac Tamponade Hypervolemia L-R shunt (ASD, VSD) LVF (CHF, MI, shock) Mitral stenosis/regurgitation ↑PVR: Acidosis, embolism, hypertension, hypoxemia, vasopressors	**Increased** Cardiac Tamponade Constrictive Pericarditis Hypervolemia LVF (CHF, MI, shock) Mitral stenosis/regurgitation Pneumothorax MV (esp. with PEEP)
Decreased Aortic Stenosis Arrhythmias Cardiac Tamponade LVF (CHF, MI, shock) Mitral Stenosis Shock	**Decreased** Hypovolemia: Absolute (loss) Relative (shock, drugs)		**Decreased** Hypovolemia: Absolute (loss) Relative (shock, drugs)	**Decreased** Hypovolemia: Absolute (loss) Relative (shock, drugs)

Some Disease Entities Causing WAVEFORM Changes

BP Waveform	CVP Waveform	PAP Waveform	
Anemia	Acute RV infarct	MV (esp. with PEEP)	Acute LV infarct
Aortic stenosis/regurgitation	Arrhythmias	Note: Most variations are	Arrhythmias
Arrhythmias	A-V Disassociation	due to technical causes.	Aortic Stenosis
Arteriosclerosis	Cardiac Tamponade		Cardiac Tamponade
Asthma (severe)	Constrictive Pericarditis		Constrictive Pericarditis
Cardiac Tamponade	Hypervolemia		Hypervolemia
Cardiomyopathy	Pulmonary Hypertension		LVF
Constrictive Pericarditis	Pulmonary Stenosis		Mitral stenosis/regur-
COPD	RVF		gitation
Essential Hypertension	Tricuspid stenosis/regurgitation		MV (esp. with PEEP)
Hyperthyroidism			
Hypovolemia			Note: Many technical
LVF			causes.
Mitral Regurgitation			
Pulmonary Embolism			
Shock			
Systemic Hypertension			

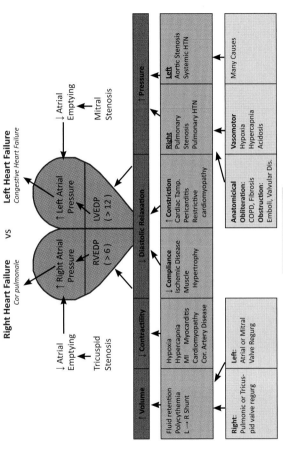

Overview of Hemodynamic Presentation in Various Disease Entities

Disease/Disorder	RR	HR	BP	PP	CO	CVP	PAP	PAWP	SVR	PVR	SvO₂
ARDS	↑	↑	↑↓	↑↓	N	N	↑	N	N	↑	↓
Cardiac Failure											
LHF	↑	↑	↑↓	↓	↓	N/↑	↑	↑	↑	↑	↓
RHF	↑	↑	↑↓	↓	↓		N	N	↑	N	↓
Cardiac Tamponade	↑	↑	N/↓	↓	N/↓	↑	↑	↑	↑	N/↑	N/↓
Cardiomyopathy	↑	↑	N/↑	↓	N/↓	↑	↑	↑	↑	N/↑	N/↓
COPD	↑	↑	N	N	N/↓	N/↑	↑	N	N/↓	↑	↓
Myocardial Infarction	N/↑	↑	↑↓	↓	N/↑	N/↑	N/↑	N/↑	↑↓	N/↑	N/↓
Pulmonary edema	↑	↑	↑	N/↓	N	N	↑	↑	↑	↑	↓
Pulmonary embolism	↑	↑	N	N	N	N	↑	N	N	↑	N/↓
Shock: Considerable Variation May Exist in all Diseases											
Anaphylactic	↑	↑	↓	↓	↓	↓	↓	↓	↓	N/↑	↓
Cardiogenic	↑	↑	↓	↓	↓	N	↑↓	↑↓	N/↑	N/↑	↓
Hypovolemic compensated	↑	↑	N/↑	N/↓	↑↓	↑↓	↑↓	↑↓	↑	↓	↓
Decompensated	↑	↑	↓	↓	↓	↓	↓	↓	↑	N/↑	↓
Neurogenic	↑↓	↓	↓	↓	N/↓	↓	↓	↓	↓	N/↑	↓
Septic (Warm)	↑	↑	N/↓	↑	N/↑	↓	↑↓	↑↓	↓	N/↑	↑
Septic (Cold)	↑	↑	↓	↓	↓	↓	↑↓	↑↓	↑↓	N/↑	↑↓
Valvular: Considerable Variation May Exist in all Diseases											
Aortic stenosis	↑	↑	↓	↓	↓	N/↑	↑	↑	↑	↑	↓
Aortic regurgitation	↑	↑	↓	↓	↓	↑	↑	↑	N/↑	↑	↓
Mitral stenosis	N/↑	N/↑	N/↓	↓	N/↓	N/↑	N/↑	N/↑	N/↑	N/↑	N/↓
Mitral regurgitation	↑	N/↑	N/↑	↓	↓	N/↑	↑	↑	N/↑	N/↑	↓

Oakes: *Hemodynamic Monitoring: A Bedside Reference Manual*, covers each of the above diseases/disorders in detail, including Definition, Etiology, Pathophysiology, Clinical Manifestations, Hemodynamic Presentation, Diagnostic Studies, and Mgmt.

9   Equations

Major categories are listed above.
All equations are alphabetically listed within each section.

EQUATIONS

Equation		Significance
Acid-Base		
Anion Gap	Normal = 12 (± 4) mEq/L	Indicates metabolic acidosis due to an increase of acid (rather than a decrease of base)
1) $AG = Na^+ - (Cl^- + HCO_3^-)$		
2) $AG = (Na^+ + K^+) - (Cl^- + HCO_3^-)$	Normal = 20 (± 4) mEq/L	
	AG = the difference between measured cations (+) and anions (−) (ie, unmeasured ions)	↑ AG = ↑ unmeasured anions (acid); **acid production:** lactate (hypoxia), ketones (diabetes) **↑acid addition:** poisons (methanol, salicylates) **↓ acid excretion:** renal failure ↓ AG = ↓ unmeasured anions: albumin
Note: When an Anion Gap Metabolic Acidosis is present, there are various methods used to calculate for additional or mixed metabolic disorders. See Oakes' *ABG Pocket Guide: Interpretation and Management* for more details.		
Base Excess (BE)	$\Delta PaCO_2$ from 40	Base deficit (BD) = − BE
1) $BE = \dfrac{\Delta PaCO_2 + \Delta pH \times 100}{2}$	ΔpH from 7.40	Accurate only in ranges of: PaCO₂: 30-50, pH 7.30-7.50
2) $BE \approx \Delta PaCO_2$	ΔHCO_3 from 24	
3) $BE \approx \Delta HCO_3 + 10 \ \Delta pH$		

ABG Pocket Guide
Interpretation and Management
Dana Oakes

Equation	Comments	Significance
Bicarbonate Correction of pH $HCO_3 = (0.2)\text{body weight} \times BD$	Corrects to pH 7.40 BD = base deficit	Used to correct for metabolic acidosis.
Henderson-Hasselbach 1) $pH = 6.1 + \log[HCO_3 / H_2CO_3]$ 2) $pH = 6.1 + \log[HCO_3 / \text{dissolved } CO_2]$ 3) $pH = 6.1 + \dfrac{\text{total } CO_2 - 0.03PaCO_2}{0.03PaCO_2}$ 4) $PaCO_2 = \dfrac{\text{total } CO_2}{0.3 \times [1 - \text{antilog}(pH - 6.1)]}$	$\text{Total } CO_2 = \dfrac{\text{volume \%}}{2.2}$	Calculation of pH or $PaCO_2$.
Rule of 8's At: pH $HCO_3 =$ 7.6 8/8 ($PaCO_2$) 7.5 6/8 ($PaCO_2$) 7.4 5/8 ($PaCO_2$) 7.3 4/8 ($PaCO_2$) 7.2 3/8 ($PaCO_2$)	Examples: when pH 7.4, $PaCO_2$ 40, $HCO_3 = 5/8\,(40) = 25$ pH 7.3, $PaCO_2$ 60, $HCO_3 = 4/8\,(60) = 30$	Estimate of HCO_3 in relation to pH and $PaCO_2$.

9-3

EQUATIONS

Equation		Significance
T40 Bicarbonate $$T40 = HCO_3 - \text{expected } \Delta HCO_3$$	HCO_3 = standard plasma Expected $\Delta HCO_3 = \dfrac{PaCO_2 - 40}{15}$	Used to find a "true" metabolic component in acute hypercapnia.
Winters Formula $PaCO_2$ predicted $= 1.54 \times HCO_3 + 8.36 \ (\pm 1)$	Measures respiratory compensation for metabolic acidosis.	$PaCO_2$ (actual) > $PaCO_2$ (pred) = mixed acidosis $PaCO_2$ (actual) < $PaCO_2$ (predicted) = respiratory alkalosis
Oxygenation		
A-a Gradient ($PA-aO_2$) ($A-aDO_2$) Alveolar- arterial O_2 tension difference	Normal = 10 - 25 mm Hg (air) = 30 - 50mm Hg (100% O_2) Increases with age and FIO_2. PaO_2 is calculated at FIO_2 0.5 breathed x 20 min to get PaO_2 > 150 (100% not used due to ↑ shunt).	Indicates efficiency of gas exchange. Normal values indicate normal shunt. Distinguishes between true shunt and V/Q mismatch. ↑ = shunt, V/Q mismatch, alveolar hypoventilation, or ↓ diffusion. > 350 mm Hg indicative of weaning failure.
1) $PA-aO_2 = PAO_2 - PaO_2$		
2) $PA-aO_2 = 140 - (PaO_2 + PaCO_2)$	ABG is drawn for $PaCO_2$ and PaO_2.	Less accurate estimate (on 21% only).
3) $PA-aO_2 / 20$	Estimate of shunt (100% O_2).	See shunt equation.

Equation		Significance
Alveolar O$_2$ Tension (Alveolar air equation) (P$_A$O$_2$)	Normal =100 mm Hg(air) = 663 mm Hg (100%, sea level)	Partial pressure of O$_2$ in alveoli. Used to determine alveolar O$_2$ tension to calculate PA-aO$_2$ gradient, a/A ratio, and % shunt.
1) P$_A$O$_2$ = ([PB - PH$_2$O] x FIO$_2$) – PaCO$_2$ x (FIO$_2$ + 1 - FIO$_2$/RE)	RE = respiratory exchange ratio (normal = 0.8)	
2) P$_A$O$_2$ = ([PB - PH$_2$O] x FIO$_2$) – PaCO$_2$ (1.25)	Short form when breathing < 100% O$_2$	
3) P$_A$O$_2$ = PIO$_2$ - PaCO$_2$ (1.25)	Short form when breathing 100% O$_2$, PIO$_2$ = (PB - PH$_2$O) x FIO$_2$	
4) P$_A$O$_2$ = 150 - PaCO$_2$ (1.25)	Estimate only on room air	
5) P$_A$O$_2$ = (FIO$_2$ x 700) - 50	Estimate only	
Arterial/Alveolar O$_2$ Tension (a/A Ratio)	Index of gas exchange function or efficiency of the lungs.	More stable than A-a gradient: A-a gradient changes with FIO$_2$, a/A remains relatively stable with FIO$_2$ changes. Changes only with PaCO$_2$ or V/Q changes.
PaO$_2$ / P$_A$O$_2$	Normal = 0.8 - 0.9 (0.75 elderly) at any FIO$_2$.	Low a/A (<0.6) = shunt, V/Q mismatch, or diffusion defect; < 0.35 indicative of weaning failure, <0.15 = refractory hypoxemia.
PaO$_2$ known / P$_A$O$_2$ calculated = PaO$_2$ desired / P$_A$O$_2$ unknown	Useful to predict PaO$_2$ when changing FIO$_2$. (See FIO$_2$ estimation equation)	Can be used to estimate shunt (See shunt equation).

EQUATIONS

EQUATIONS

Equation		Significance
Arterial-(mixed)Venous O_2 Content Difference $(Ca-\bar{v}O_2)$ $CaO_2 - C\bar{v}O_2 = Ca-\bar{v}O_2$	Difference between arterial and mixed venous O_2 contents. Normal = 4.2 - 5.0 mL/dL (vol%)	Represents O_2 consumption by tissue and estimate of cardiac output. $\uparrow = \downarrow CO$ or $\uparrow$ metabolism. $\downarrow = \uparrow CO$ or $\downarrow$ metabolism.
Arterial-(mixed)Venous O_2 Tension Difference $(Pa-\bar{v}O_2,$ or $a-\bar{v}DO_2)$ $PaO_2 - P\bar{v}O_2 = Pa-\bar{v}O_2$	Normal = 60 mm Hg	Difference between arterial and mixed venous O_2 tensions.
Arterial CO_2 tension (PaCO2) $PaCO2 = \dfrac{\dot{V}CO_2}{\dot{V}A}$	Normal = 35-45 mm Hg	
FIO2 Estimation 1) Using a/A ratio: $PAO_2 = PaO_2$ desired $/$ a/A ratio 2) Using alveolar O_2 tension: $FIO_2 = PAO_2 + (PaCO_2 / 0.8) / (PB-H_2O)$ 3) Using A-a gradient: $FIO_2 = PA-aO_2 +$ desired $PaO_2 / .760$ 4) Using P/F Ratio: PaO_2 should be: $\dfrac{5\,PaO_2}{1\,FIO_2}$ 5) Estimate: $FIO_2 = PaO_2 / 500$	Figured at any FIO_2 Need $\uparrow FIO_2$ x 20 minutes	Used to estimate the FIO_2 needed to achieve a desired PaO_2 or the PaO_2 that will be achieved at any given FIO_2. $\dfrac{Current\ PaO_2}{Current\ FIO_2} = \dfrac{Desired\ PaO_2}{New\ FIO_2}$ New $FIO_2 = PaO_2$ desired $+ PaCO_2$ desired $/ (PaO_2/PAO_2) / (PB - H_2O)$

Equation	Normal Value	Significance
O_2 Consumption (Demand) ($\dot{V}O_2$) $\dot{V}O_2 = CO \times (CaO_2 - C\bar{v}O2) \times 10$ $= CO \times Ca\text{-}\bar{v}O_2 \times 10$	Normal = 200 - 250 mL/min	Volume of O_2 consumed (utilized) by the body tissues per min. Index of metabolic level and CO. $\uparrow\dot{V}O_2 = \uparrow$metabolism or CO; $\downarrow\dot{V}O_2 = \downarrow$metabolism or CO
O_2 Consumption Index ($\dot{V}O_2I$) $\dot{V}O_2I = CI \times Ca\text{-}\bar{v}O_2 \times 10$	$\dot{V}O_2I = \dot{V}O_2/BSA$ $= 110\text{-}165\ mL/min/m^2$	O_2 consumption per body size.
O_2 Content 1) Arterial $CaO_2 = (Hgb \times 1.36) \times SaO_2 +$ $(PaO_2 \times 0.0031)$	Normal = 15-24 mL/dL (vol%) Both 1.36 and 1.39 are considered correct. Hgb = gm %	Total amount of O_2 in arterial blood (combined plus dissolved).
2) Venous (mixed) $C\bar{v}O_2 = (Hgb \times 1.36) \times S\bar{v}O_2 +$ $(P\bar{v}O_2 \times 0.0031)$ $= \dot{V}O_2/CO$	Normal = 12-15 mL/dL (vol%) $P\bar{v}O_2$ = pressure in mixed venous blood obtained from pulmonary artery.	Total amount of O_2 in mixed venous blood (combined plus dissolved).
3) Pulmonary capillary CcO_2	See shunt equation.	SaO_2 and $S\bar{v}O_2$ obtained from oximeter or oxyheme dissociation curve.

Equation	Significance
O₂ Delivery (Supply, Transport) ($\dot{D}O_2$) $\dot{D}O_2 = CO \times CaO_2 \times 10$	Normal = 750-1000 mL/min Quantity of O_2 delivered to the body tissues per minute. Requires CO determination.	↑O_2 transport =↑CO +/or ↑CaO_2 ↓O_2 transport =↓CO +/or ↓CaO_2 10 = conversion factor to mL/min
O₂ Delivery Index ($\dot{D}O_2I$) $\dot{D}O_2I = CI \times CaO_2 \times 10$	$\dot{D}O_2I = \dot{D}O_2 / BSA$ = 500-600 mL/min/m² O_2 delivery per body size.
O₂ Extraction Ratio (O₂ ER) $O_2\ ER = \dfrac{O_2\ consumption\ (demand)}{O_2\ delivery\ (supply)}$ $= \dfrac{\dot{V}O_2}{\dot{D}O_2} \times 100$ $= \dfrac{Ca\text{-}\bar{v}O_2}{CaO_2}$	Normal = 25 % Amount of O_2 extracted and consumed by the body tissues, relative to the amount delivered. Estimate $= \dfrac{Sa\text{-}\bar{v}O_2}{SaO_2}$	Indicator of O_2 supply/demand balance. ↑ratio = ↓FO₂ +/or ↑ O_2 transport ↓ ratio = ↑O₂+/or ↓ O_2 transport
O₂ Index (OI)	$OI = (\bar{P}aw \times FIO_2 \times 100) / PaO_2$	> 40 = severe respiratory distress with high mortality; 20 - 25 = mortality > 50%
O₂ Reserve $O_2\ Reserve = \dot{D}O_2 - \dot{V}O_2$	Normal = 750 mL/min $= CO \times C\bar{v}O_2 \times 10$	Venous O_2 supply: O_2 supply minus O_2 demand

Equation		Significance
O2 Saturation (mixed venous) (SvO₂) $SvO_2 = SaO_2 - \dot{V}O_2/\dot{D}O_2$ $= SaO_2 - Sa-\bar{v}O_2$	Normal = 75 % (60-80 %)	Percent of hemoglobin in mixed venous blood, saturated with O_2,
O2 Saturation (SaO₂) $SaO_2 = HbO_2/Total\ Hb \times 100$	Normal - 95-100% HbO_2 = Oxyhemoglobin Content	% of Hemoglobin available that is carrying Oxygen
P/F Ratio (Oxygenation Ratio) PaO_2 / FIO_2	Normal = 400 – 500 (regardless of FIO_2) What PaO_2 Should Be: $\dfrac{5\ PaO_2}{1\ FIO_2\%}$	< 300 indicative of ALI < 200 = ARDS
Predicted PaO₂ (based on age)	$PaO_2 = 110 - \frac{1}{2}$ age	
Respiratory Index (RI) $PA-aO_2 / PaO_2$	Normal = < 1.0	1.0- 5.0 = V/Q mismatch > 5.0 = refractory hypoxemia due to physiol. shunt

Equation		Significance
Respiratory Quotient (RQ, RE, RR) (Exchange ratio)		RQ = ratio of CO_2 produced to O_2 consumed (internal respiration). RE represents the amount of O_2/CO_2 exchange in the lungs per minute (external respiration). $RE = RQ$ in steady state condition.
1) $RQ = \dfrac{\dot{V}CO_2}{\dot{V}O_2}$	Volume CO_2 produced/min / Volume O_2 consumed/min	
	Normal = 200 / 250 = 0.8	
2) $RQ = \dot{V}_E \times \dfrac{F\bar{E}\,CO_2 - FCO_2}{FiO_2 - F\bar{E}\,O_2}$		
3) $RQ = \dfrac{F\bar{E}\,CO_2}{FIO_2 - F\bar{E}\,O_2}$		
Ventilation/Perfusion Index (VQI) $VQI = \dfrac{1 - SaO_2}{1 - S\bar{v}O_2}$	Normal = 0.8	Combines assessment of SaO_2 and $S\bar{v}O_2$ to estimate venous admixture. Correlates well with $\dot{Q}s/\dot{Q}t$.
Ventilation		
Alveolar Ventilation ($\dot{V}_A$)	Normal = 4 - 6 L/min	The volume of inspired air which participates in gas exchange per minute.
1) $\dot{V}_A = \dot{V}_E - \dot{V}_D$	$\dot{V}_ECO_2 = \dot{V}_E$ measured $\times$ F$\bar{E}$ CO_2 calculated or measured	
2) $\dot{V}_A = (V_T - V_{Dphys}) \times f$	F$\bar{E}$ $CO_2 = P\bar{E}$ CO_2 measured / PB – PH$_2$O	
3) $\dot{V}_A = (\dot{V}_ECO_2/PaCO_2) \times 863$	863 = correction factor if in milliliters, (0.863 = if in liters).	Used to calculate the ideal alveolar ventilation needed to maintain a desired $PaCO_2$.
4) Ideal $\dot{V}_A = (\dot{V}_ECO_2 / PaCO_2$ desired$) \times 863$	Estimated $\dot{V}_ECO_2 = 3mL/kg/min$	
5) $\dot{V}_A \times PaCO_2$ known = $\dot{V}_A \times$ $PaCO_2$ desired		

Equation	Comments	Significance
Alveolar Volume (V_A) 1) $V_A = \dot{V}_A / f$ 2) $V_A = V_T - V_D$ 3) $V_A = 2 \times IBW$ (lbs) 4) $V_A = 2/3\ V_T$	Estimate Estimate (normal)	The volume of each breath that participates in gas exchange.
Deadspace Ventilation ($\dot{V}_D$) 1) $\dot{V}_{Dphys} = V_{Dphys} \times f$ 2) $\dot{V}_{Dphys} = \dot{V}_E - \dot{V}_A$ 3) $\dot{V}_{Dphys} = \left(\dfrac{PaCO_2 - PECO_2}{PaCO_2} \right) \times \dot{V}_E$ 4) $\dot{V}_{Dphys} = \dot{V}_D/V_T \times \dot{V}_E$	Normal = $1/3\ \dot{V}_E$	The volume of wasted air (not participating in gas exchange) per minute.
Deadspace Volume (V_D) 1) $V_D = V_T - V_A$ 2) $V_D = \dot{V}_E - \dfrac{\dot{V}_A}{f}$ 3) $V_{Dphys} = V_{Danat} + V_{Dalv} +$ $V_{Dmech} + V_{Dcomp} = $ total V_D	Normal = $1/3\ V_T$ V_{Danat} = anatomical V_D (1 mL/lb IBW; 0.5 mL/lb with ET tube or trach) V_{Dalv} = alveolar V_D V_{Dmech} = mechanical (10mL/inch) V_{Dcomp} = tubing compliance loss	The volume of wasted air (not participating in gas exchange) per breath (V > Q). $\uparrow V_{Dalv} = \downarrow$ CO, pulmonary vasoconstriction, pulmonary embolus

Equation		Significance
Deadspace / Tidal Volume Ratio (V_D /V_T Ratio)	Normal = 0.33 $\frac{(150\ V_D)}{(450\ V_T)}$	Used to measure the portion of V_T not participating in gas exchange (wasted ventilation).
1) Bohr Equation: $\frac{V_Dphys = PaCO_2 - P\overline{E}\ CO_2}{V_T \qquad PaCO_2}$ $\frac{V_Danat = PetCO_2 - P\overline{E}\ CO_2}{V_T \qquad PetCO_2}$	$P\overline{E}\ CO_2$ = mixed expired Normal = 0.33 (no ABG required) Pet = end tidal	$V_D/V_T > 0.5$ is indicative of respiratory failure. Many lung diseases (atelectasis, pneumonia, pulmonary edema, emboli, etc.) can exhibit changes in V_D (i.e., V_DalV) without corresponding changes in $PaCO_2$.
2) Estimate: V_Dphys / V_T = ($\dot{V}_E$ actual / $\dot{V}_E$ predicted) x ($PaCO_2$ actual / 40) x 0.33	This equation is quite accurate. No mixed expired sample required.	
Minute Ventilation ($\dot{V}_E$) (Minute Volume)	Normal = 5 - 7 L/min.	The total air in or out of the lungs in one minute.
1) $\dot{V}_E = V_T$ x f 2) $\dot{V}_E = \dot{V}_A + \dot{V}_D$ 3) $\dot{V}_E = 1/PaCO_2$	Changing f is often preferred to changing V_T (due to altering V_D/V_T ratio).	Used to calculate the $\dot{V}_E$ needed to maintain a desired $PaCO_2$.
4) New $\dot{V}_E = \dot{V}_E$ current x $PaCO_2$ current/ $PaCO_2$ desired 5)$PaCO_2$ desired x $\dot{V}_E$ needed = $PaCO_2$ current x $\dot{V}_E$ current 6) Nomogram (See next page)	$\dot{V}_A$ = effective alveolar ventilation $\dot{V}_D$ = physiological deadspace	Change rate to change $\dot{V}_E$, changing V_T may alter the V_D/V_T ratio.

Equation	Comments	Significance
Ventilation/Perfusion Ratio (V̇/Q̇ Ratio) $\dot{V}_A/\dot{Q}c = \dfrac{(C\overline{v}CO_2 - CaCO_2) \times 8.63}{PaCO_2}$	Normal = 4L/min = 0.8 5L/min Ratio of minute alveolar ventilation to minute capillary blood flow. Represents external respiration.	Ratio changes represent the degree and type of respiratory imbalances. ↓ Ratio (↓V/Q) = atelectasis, COPD, pneumonia, pneumothorax, N-M disorders, etc. ↑ Ratio (V/↑Q) = shock, pulmonary emboli, cor pulmonale, PPV.

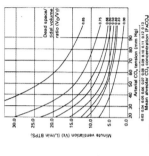

Nomogram to estimate minute ventilation required to maintain a given PaCO2 when VD/VT is known:

To obtain the require minute ventilation to achieve a given PaCO2, the minute ventilation is plotted against the PaCO2 (measured simultaneously) and the VD/VT ratio is read on the isopleth that corresponds to the intersection. The isopleth is then followed to the desired PaCO2 and the corresponding minute ventilation read off the vertical axis.

For example: A patient with a VE of 5L and a PaCO2 of 60 mmHg has an estimated VD/VT ratio of 0.40. To achieve a desired PaCO2 of 40 mmHg, follow the 0.40 isopleth up to correspond to the PaCO2 of 40 on the horizontal axis. Then read the appropriate minute ventilation of about 8L/min off the vertical axis.

9-13

Equation		Significance
Ventilator Calculations		
Ventilator Flow $\dot{V} = \dot{V}_E \times RFF$ or $\dot{V} = \dot{V}_E \times 1/TI\%$	RFF = ratio flow factor = I + E Example: I:E ratio = 1:3, RFF = 4	Used to calculate proper flow to deliver a V_T in a given T_I.
Ventilator Rate Needed for Desired $PaCO_2$ New rate = current rate x $\dfrac{PaCO_2}{\text{desired } PaCO_2}$	Desired $\dot{V}_E$ = $\dfrac{\text{Current } PaCO_2 \times \text{ Current } \dot{V}_E}{\text{desired } PaCO_2}$	This equation holds presuming a steady metabolic rate, stable or no spontaneous breathing, and no change in other ventilator parameters, or Vomech.
Mechanics		
Airway Occlusion Pressure (P0.1)	Normal = < 2 cm H_2O Change in airway pressure at 0.1 sec after beginning inspiration against an occluded airway. Used to assess ventilatory drive and demand. Indicative of ventilatory demand.	↑ P0.1 = ↑ patient workload +/or drive (possible inadequate ventilator support). ↓ P0.1 = ↓ patient workload +/or drive (possible excessive ventilator support). > 4 - 6 cm H_2O is indicative of weaning failure. (See PImax) Although actual value is negative, it is reported as a positive.

Equation	Comments	Significance
Airway Resistance (Raw) 1) $R = \Delta P / \dot{V}$ 2) $Raw = Pmouth - Palv / \dot{V}_I$ 3) $Raw = PIP - Pplat / \dot{V}_I$ 4) $Raw = Cdyn - Cstat$ (see below)	Normal = 0.5 - 2.5 cm H_2O/L/sec @ 0.5 L/sec (30 L/min) ET tube = 4 - 8 cm H_2O/L/sec $\dot{V}_I$ = inspiratory flow in L/sec; square wave flow pattern (use 30 L/min if comparing with norm).	Represents frictional resistance of airflow (80%) and tissue motion (20%). $Raw = 1/r^4$ ↑ airflow resistance = airway collapse, edema, bronchospasm, secretions, ET tube etc. ↑ tissue resistance = pulmonary edema, fibrosis, pneumonia, etc. (see Ch 7). > 5 cm H_2O/L/sec may = wean failure.
Clinical Note: A quick estimate of Raw: = P_{TA} (transairway pressure) = PIP - Pplat ↑P_{TA} = ↑Raw ↓P_{TA} = ↓Raw	↑PIP + ↑Pplat (P_{TA} constant) = ↓Cstat ↑PIP + same Pplat (↑P_{TA}) = ↑Raw ↓PIP + ↓Pplat (P_{TA} constant) = ↑Cstat ↓PIP + same Pplat (↓P_{TA}) = ↓Raw	Pressure support is used primarily to overcome airway resistance of circuit and ET tube. Appropriate PS level can be estimated as PTA (i.e., PIP - Pplat). Note: By convention Raw refers to inspiratory Raw. Expiratory Raw may be determined by PIP - PEEP / $\dot{V}$expir and is typically > inspiratory Raw.

EQUATIONS

Equation		Significance
Compliance (C) $C = \Delta V / \Delta P$ $C_{LT} = C_L + C_{cw}$ $= \Delta V / Palv - PB$	Normal = 70 - 100 mL/cm H2O Total compliance is referred to as C_{LT} (lung + thorax) or C_{rs} (respiratory system). C_L = lung compliance C_{cw} = chest wall (thorax) compliance	Represents the ease of distention of the lungs and thorax. Includes elastic, functional, and tissue viscous resistance. Ideal = 100mL/ cm H2O Lungs and chest wall each = 200 mL/ cm H2O.
$C_L = \Delta V / Palv - Ppl$ $C_{cw} = \Delta V / Ppl - PB$		P_B = barometric pressure; Ppl = pleural pressure Palv = alveolar pressure

9-16

Equation	How to Measure	Significance
Static Compliance (Cstat) **How To Measure** $Cstat = V_T - V_{tubing} / Pplat - PEEP$ Pplat = the pressure needed to maintain lung inflation during zero airflow. It is measured by using either an inspiratory hold or temporarily occluding the exhalation port until pressure stabilizes (approx 1 - 4 sec). $PEEP = PEEP_E + PEEP_I$ Clinical Note: In VV, a ↓Cstat results in an ↑PIP and ↑Pplat (V_T constant). In PV, a ↓Cstat results in a ↓V_T (PIP and Pplat constant).	Normal = 70 - 100 mL/cm H2O V_{tubing} = volume loss in tubing due to circuit compliance $V_{tubing} = CF$ (tubing compliance factor) $\times$ $P_{gradient}$ (Pplat - PEEP) CF must be determined for each patient-ventilator setup (normals range from 1.5 - 5.0 mL/cm H2O). It is either calculated by newer ventilators or manually by: setting V_T to 200 mL, triggering the ventilator, occluding the patient wye, and observing PIP. $CF = V_T (200) / PIP$ (Pplat can be used in place of PIP). $V_{tubing} = (V_T (200) / PIP) \times (Pplat - PEEP)$	Represents the combination of lung elasticity and chest wall recoil. Usually measured while on MV. ↓ Cstat = ↓ lung elasticity or ↓ chest wall recoil. ↑ Cstat = ↑ lung elasticity or ↑ chest wall recoil. For conditions causing ↑ or ↓ Cstat, see Oakes' *Ventilator Management* book. Trend changes in Cstat and Cdyn are more significant in interpreting lung conditions than single measurements. A Cstat ≤ 25- 33 mL/cm H2O is indicative of weaning failure. Cstat can also be used to determine optimal PEEP.

9-17

Equation		Significance
Dynamic Compliance (Cdyn)	Normal = 40 - 70 mL/cm H₂O	Represents the combination of static lung compliance (Cstat) and airway resistance (Raw).
How To Measure Cdyn = Vt - Vtubing / PIP - PEEP Usually measured while on MV.	Vtubing = CF x (PIP - PEEP) (See Cstat above to determine CF) PEEP = PEEP₁ + PEEP	For conditions causing ↑ or ↓Cdyn, see Cstat (above) Trend changes in Cstat and Cdyn are more significant in interpreting lung conditions than single measurements.

Clinical Notes:

	↑Cdyn (same Cstat) = ↓Raw ↓Cdyn (same Cstat) = ↑Raw
In VV, a↓ Cdyn results in an↑PIP (Vt constant). In VV, a ↓PIP (Vt constant) = improved Cstat or Raw or a leak.	↑Cdyn (with same↓ in Cstat) = ↑Cstat ↓Cdyn (with same ↓ in Cstat) = ↓Cstat
In PV, a ↓Cdyn results in a ↓Vt (PIP constant). In PV, an ↑Vt (PIP constant) = improved Cstat or Raw.	↑Cdyn (with partial ↑ in Cstat) = ↓Raw and ↑Cstat ↓Cdyn (with partial ↓ in Cstat) = ↑Raw and ↓Cstat

Equation	Significance	
Equation of Motion $Pawo = V/C + (Raw \times \dot{V})$	Elastic components of respiratory system: $P = V/C$ $V = P \times C$ $C = V/P$ Resistive components of respiratory system: $P = Raw \times \dot{V}$ $\dot{V} = P/Raw$ $Raw = P/\dot{V}$	At any moment the airway opening pressure (Pawo) must exactly balance the opposing lung and chest wall expansion forces. $P, \dot{V}, V$ can be controlled by the clinician. In VV: Set $\dot{V}$: P varies with Raw Set V: P varies with C In PV: Set P: $\dot{V}$ varies with Raw Set P: V varies with C
Maximal Inspiratory Pressure (Pimax) (MIP, NIP) Two methods: Marini #1- total occlusion @ end-exhalation Marini #2- total occlusion @ below FRC	The maximal inspiratory effort (pressure) generated against an occluded airway (approx 20 sec). Normal < 20 cm H_2O (i.e., < - 20 cm H_2O) Although actual value is negative, it is reported as a positive.	Indicative of the capability of the inspiratory muscles. (See P0.1 above) P0.1 / Pimax = demand / capability = predictive weaning index ≤ 0.9 indicative of weaning failure Prior to start of test patient should be actively breathing (remove vent support). Remove PEEPe and PEEPi. Respiratory muscles should not be fatigued.

9-19

Equation		Significance
Mean Airway Pressure ($\overline{P}aw$) $$\overline{P}aw = \frac{(T_I \times PIP) + (T_E \times PEEP)}{Ttot}$$ $$\overline{P}aw = (PIP - PEEP) \times T_I/Ttot + PEEP$$	Average airway pressure during several breathing cycles.	$\overline{P}aw = ([P_{IA} + \frac{1}{2} PA] - PEEP) \times T_I/Ttot + PEEP$ Note: Should always be less than CVP (1 cm H2O = 0.735 mmHg)
Rapid - Shallow Breathing Index (RSBI) $RSBI = f / V_T$ or $f^2 / \dot{V}_E$	Measure f and V_T (in liters) while off the ventilator. Normal = < 100	Has proven to be one of the best predictive indices for weaning. > 105 is indicative of weaning failure
Time Constant (TC) $TC = Raw \times Cstat$ $TC = \Delta P/\dot{V} \times \Delta V/\Delta P$ **Note:** TC generally refers to inspiratory TC. Expiratory TC may be much longer than inspiratory TC in COPD.	1TC = 63% 2TC = 87% 3TC = 95% 4TC = 98% 5TC = 99% % = % of V_T entering lungs within each TC period. Normal TC = 0.2 sec Normal T_I = 3 - 4TC = 3 or 4 x 0.2 sec = 0.6 - 0.8 sec	TC (inspir) indicates alveolar filling time. ↑TC (> 0.2 sec) is usually indicative of ↑Raw (but may be ↑C$_{LT}$). ↓TC (< 0.2 sec) is usually indicative of ↓C$_{LT}$ (but may be ↓Raw). TC(expir) indicates alveolar emptying time. < 3 TCexpir will generally result in air-trapping. TCexpir may be approximated with a F-V loop.

Equation		Significance
Vital Capacity (VC)	Normal is 60-80 mL/kg	< 60 mL/kg indicates general restr. process > 10 mL/kg is needed for effective deep breathing and cough. < 10 mL/kg = impending respiratory failure
Work of Breathing (WOB) $W = \int p \times V$ $WOB / min (W) = WOB \times f$ $WOB / liter = W / \dot{V}_E$ $WOB\ total = WOB\ patient + WOB\ vent$	The energy (pressure gradient) required to take a breath. Normal = 0.6 - 1.0 j (1j = 0.1 kg.m) $W / \dot{V}_I$ closely reflects abnormal pulmonary mechanics.	Intrinsic WOB = energy required to overcome patient's elastic and resistive forces. Extrinsic WOB = energy required to overcome added extrinsic systems
Weaning Equations		
CROP $CROP = Cdyn \times (PaO_2/PAO_2) \times PImax / rate$	C = compliance R = rate O = oxygenation P = pressure	< 13 mL/breath/min indicative of weaning failure.
Simplified Weaning Index $SWI = f (mech) \times (PIP - PEEP / PImax) \times (PaCO_2 / 40)$	Normal = < 9 min	Simplified version of weaning index (WI). Less accurate than WI, but quick and easy. > 11 min indicative of weaning failure
P0.1 / PImax and RSBI (f /Vт): See above		

EQUATIONS

Equation	Significance
Perfusion/Hemodynamic Monitoring	
Cardiac Index (CI) CI = CO/BSA	More precise measure of pump efficiency than CO. CI 1.8 - 2.5 = moderate cardiac disease CI < 1.8 = severe cardiac disease Cardiac output per body size. Normal = 2.5 - 4.4 L/min/m^2 BSA (See Pg 9-28)
Cardiac Output (CO or $\dot{Q}_T$) CO = SV x HR	Amount of blood ejected from heart per minute. Indicator of pump efficiency and a determinant of tissue perfusion. Normal = 4-8 L/min (at rest) See Fick equation below & Oakes' *Hemodynamic Monitoring: A Bedside Reference Manual* for more information.
Coronary Artery Perfusion Pressure (CPP or CAPP) CPP = MAP - PAWP = BPdia - PAWP	Driving pressure of coronary blood flow. Normal = 60-80 mm Hg
Fick Equation $\dot{V}O_2$ = CO x Ca-$\bar{v}O_2$	Method of measuring cardiac output. Fick estimate: CO = 125 x BSA / Ca-$\bar{v}O_2$ See Oakes' *Hemodynamic Monitoring: A Bedside Reference Manual* for more info.

Equation	Constants	Significance
Left Ventricular Stroke Work (LVSW) $LVSW = (\overline{BP} - PAWP) \times SV \times 0.0136$	Normal = 60-80 gm/m/beat	Measure of pumping function of left ventricle (LV contractility).
Left Ventricular Stroke Work Index (LVSWI) $LVSWI = (\overline{BP} - PAWP) \times SVI \times 0.0136$	Normal = 40-75 gm/m/beat/m²	Measure of pumping function of left ventricle (LV contractility) / body size.
Mean Arterial Blood Pressure $(\overline{BP}, MAP)$ $\overline{BP} = 1/3\ PP + BPdia$ $= \dfrac{BP_{sys} + 2BP_{dia}}{3}$	Normal = 93 mm Hg (70-105)	Average driving force of systemic circulation. Determined by cardiac output and total peripheral resistance.
Mean Pulmonary Artery Pressure $(\overline{PAP}, PAMP)$ $\overline{PAP} = 1/3\ pulmPP + PADP$ $= \dfrac{PASP + 2PADP}{3}$	Normal = 10 - 15 mm Hg	Average driving force of blood from the right heart to left heart.
Pulmonary Vascular Resistance (PVR) $PVR = \dfrac{PAMP - PAWP}{CO} \times 80$	Normal = 20-250 dynes•sec•cm⁻⁵ = 0.25-2.5 units (mm Hg/L/min) E.g. $\dfrac{14\ mm\ Hg - 5\ mm\ Hg}{5\ L/min}$ = 1.8 units	Resistance to RV ejection of blood into pulmonary vasculature. Indicator of RV afterload. mm Hg/L/min x 80 = dynes•sec•cm⁻⁵

Equation	Value	Significance
Pulmonary Vascular Resistance Index (PVRI) $PVRI = \dfrac{PAMP - PAWP \times 80}{CI}$	Normal = 35-350 dynes•sec•cm^{-5}/ m^2	PVR related to body size.
Pulse Pressure (PP) $PP = BPsys - BPdia$	Normal = 40 mm Hg (20-80)	Difference between BP systolic and BP diastolic.
Rate Pressure Product (RPP) $RPP = BPsys \times HR$	Normal = < 12,000 mm Hg/min	Indirect determinant of M$\dot{V}O_2$.
Right Ventricular Stroke Work (RVSW) = $(PAMP - CVP) \times SV \times 0.0136$	Normal = 10-15 gm/m/beat	Measure of pumping function of right ventricle (RV contractility).
Right Ventricular Stroke Work Index (RVSW) = $(PAMP - CVP) \times SVI \times 0.0136$	Normal = 4-12 gm/m/beat/m^2 = RVSW / BSA	Measure of pumping function of right ventricle (RV contractility) / body size.

Equation		Significance
Shunt Equation $(\dot{Q}_s/\dot{Q}_t)$		Indicates ratio of shunted blood $(\dot{Q}_s)$ (blood not participating in gas exchange) to total cardiac output $(\dot{Q}_t)$.
1) Classical $\dot{Q}_s/\dot{Q}_t = \dfrac{CcO_2 - CaO_2}{Cc-\bar{v}O_2}$	Normal = 2-5%. CcO_2 = pulmonary capillary blood O_2 content ("ideal") at 100% saturated with alveolar O_2. Cannot be sampled. CcO_2 = (Hgb x 1.34) SaO_2 + (PAO$_2$ x 0.003)	$\dot{Q}_s = \dot{Q}_t - \dot{Q}_c$ $\dot{Q}_s = \dot{Q}sphys = \dot{Q}sanat + \dot{Q}scap$ Indicator or efficiency of pulm system: < 10% = normal lungs 10-20% = minimal effect 20-30% = significant pulm disease > 30% = life-threatening
2) Clinical $\dot{Q}_s/\dot{Q}_t = \dfrac{PA\text{-}aO_2 \times 0.003}{Ca\text{-}\bar{v}O_2 + PA\text{-}aO_2 \times 0.003}$	Less accurate/easier. Perform breathing ↑FIO$_2$ (50% preferred over 100% due to ↑shunting from alveolar collapse) x 20 minutes.	Clinical equation assumes Hgb 100% saturated (PaO$_2$ > 150). If PaO$_2$ < 150, then must use classical shunt equation.
3) Estimate $\dot{Q}_s/\dot{Q}_t = \dfrac{PA\text{-}aO_2 \times 0.003}{3.5 + PA\text{-}aO_2 \times 0.003}$		Ca-$\bar{v}O_2$ can be assumed if a mixed venous sample cannot be obtained: 4.5 - 5% in patients with good CO and perfusion. 3.5% in critically ill patients.
4) Estimates $\dot{Q}_s/\dot{Q}_t = \dfrac{PA\text{-}aO_2}{20}$ $\dot{Q}_s/\dot{Q}_t$ = 5% per every 100 mm Hg below expected	5%/100 mm Hg (2%/50 mm Hg) Most accurate when breathing 100% O$_2$. Plus normal 2-5%. Estimate good until PaO$_2$ < 100 mm Hg.	Estimate: PaO$_2$/FIO$_2$ > 300 = < 15% shunt 200 - 300 = 15 - 20%; < 200 = > 20% shunt

EQUATIONS

9-25

Equation		Significance
Stroke Volume (SV) $SV = CO/HR \times 1000$	Normal = 60-120 mL/beat	Amount of blood ejected by either ventricle per contraction.
Stroke Volume Index (SVI) $SVI = CO/HR \times 1000 / BSA$	Normal = 35-75 mL/beat/m²	Relates SV to body size.
Systemic Vascular Resistance (SVR) $SVR = \dfrac{\overline{BP} - CVP}{CO} \times 80$	Normal = 800-1600 dynes•sec•cm⁻⁵ = 10-20 units (mm Hg/L/min) E.g. $\dfrac{93 \text{ mm Hg} - 3 \text{ mm Hg}}{5 \text{ L/min}} = 18$ units	Resistance to LV ejection of blood into systemic circulation. Indicator of LV afterload. mm Hg/L/min x 80 = dynes•sec•cm⁻⁵
Systemic Vascular Resistance Index (SVRI) $SVRI = \dfrac{\overline{BP} - CVP}{CI} \times 80$	Normal = 1400-2600 dynes•sec•cm⁻⁵ / m²	SVR per body size.
Patient Calculations		
Body Surface Area (BSA) $BSA \ (m^2) = (Ht \ (cm)^{0.725}) \times (Wt \ (kg)^{0.425}) \times .007184$	BSA (m²) = (4 x Kg) + 7 / Kg + 90	Used to determine cardiac index and other hemodynamic parameters. Relates parameters to body size. Kg = 2.2 lbs

Equation	Comments	Significance
Ideal Body Weight (IBW) Kg = 2.2 lbs	**SHORTCUT:** Male: 106 lbs for 5 ft tall. Add 6 lbs/in above 5 ft. **ARDS NET:** Wt [kg] = 50.0 + 0.91 (Ht [cm] - 152.4)	Female: 100 lbs for 5 ft tall. Add 5 lbs/in above 5 ft. Wt [kg] = 45.5 + 0.91 (Ht [cm] - 152.4)
Pulmonary Function (Bedside)		
% Predicted	$\dfrac{\text{Actual}}{\text{Predicted}} \times 100$	
% Change	$\dfrac{\text{Post Value - Pre value}}{\text{Pre Value}} \times 100$	
Miscellaneous		
ATPS to BTPS Vol BTPS = Vol ATPS x factor	See Appendix	Correction of lung volumes measured at room temp to body temp.
Fick's Law of Diffusion Diffusion = Area x diffusion coefficient x $\dfrac{\Delta P}{\text{Thickness}}$		Gas diffusion rate across the lung membrane.

EQUATIONS

9-27

EQUATIONS

Equation	Comments	Significance
Gas Laws Dalton's Law: Boyle's Law: Charles' Law: Gay-Lussac's Law: Combined Gas Law:	$Total\ P = P1+P2+P3$, etc. $P1 \times V1 = P2 \times V2$ $V1/T1 = V2/T2$ $P1/T1 = P2/T2$ $P1 \times V1/T1 = P2 \times V2/T2$	P and V are inversely related (T constant) V and T are directly related (P constant) P and T are directly related (V constant)
Graham's Law of Diffusion Coefficient	Diffusion coefficient = $\dfrac{solubility\ coefficient}{\sqrt{gmw}}$	Rate of gas diffusion is inversely proportional to the square root of its gram molecular weight.
Helium/Oxygen (He/O₂) Flow Conversion and Duration	80% He / 20% O₂: actual flow = flow x 1.8 70% He / 30% O₂ = flow x 1.6 60% He / 40% O₂ = flow x 1.4 Duration Factor (see next page, O2)	Conversion is used when an O₂ flow meter is used to measure flow. Used in patients with obstructive disorders.
Law of LaPlace	$P = 2ST / r$	P = pressure (dynes/cm²); r = radius (cm) ST = surface tension (dynes/cm)

Equation	Comments	Significance
Oxygen Blending Ratios $100 \xleftarrow{\text{FIO}_2 \text{ desired}} 21$ air units ——— O2 units	Select desired FIO$_2$: Subtract 100 - FIO$_2$ = air units Subtract FIO$_2$ - 20 = O$_2$ units	To find air/O$_2$ ratio for desired FIO$_2$: Air units/O$_2$ units = air/O$_2$ ratio E.g: 40% O$_2$ desired $\quad$ 100 - 40 = 60 = 3 $\quad$ 40 - 20 = 20 $\quad$ 1
Oxygen Duration Times **Duration of a Cylinder** Time (min) = $\dfrac{\text{Pcyl} \times \text{CF}}{\text{Flow (L/min)}}$	Pcyl = total pressure in cylinder (psi) – 500 psi (reserve) CF = conversion factor (L/psi) $= \dfrac{(\text{ft}^3 \text{ of cyl}) \times 28.3\ \text{L/ft}^3}{\text{max Pcyl}}$ **Heliox H Culinder Duration Factor:** 2.50 **O2/CO2 H Cylinder Duration Factor:** 3.84	Used to calculate how long a cylinder of O2 gas will last. 500 psi equals reserve.

Size (Aluminum)	PSIG	factor
A	2216	0.035
B	2216	0.068
D	2015	0.16
E	2015	0.28
		0.23
		0.35
G		2.41
H/K	2265	3.14
M	2216	1.65

EQUATIONS

Equation		Significance
Duration of a Liquid System	Liquid weight is known: Duration time (min) = $$\frac{344 \text{ l/lb} \times \text{liquid weight (lb)}}{\text{O}_2 \text{ flow (L/min)}}$$ 1 L liquid = 860 L gas Liquid Wt = Total Wt - Cylinder Wt	Gauge fraction is known: Duration time (min) = $$\frac{\text{Liquid capacity (L)} \times 860 \times \text{gauge fraction}}{\text{O}_2 \text{ flow (L/min)}}$$ Does not account for evaporative loss.
Oxygen Entrainment Ratios $$TF = \text{O}_2 \text{ flow} \times \frac{0.79}{FIO_2 - 0.21}$$ Mixture $=$ O$_2$ $+$ air $$FIO_2 = \frac{0.79}{\frac{TF}{\text{O}_2 \text{ Flow}}} + 0.21$$	TF = total flow in liters (O$_2$ + air) Mixture $=$ O$_2$ $+$ air $(FIO_2)(Flow) = (1.0)(O_2 \text{ Flow}) +$ $(0.21)(\text{air Flow})$	Determines total flows, entrained flows, or O$_2$ percent when air and O$_2$ are entrained together. See O$_2$ blending ratio above.
Poiseuille's Law $$\dot{V} = \frac{\Delta P \cdot 4\pi}{\mu L 8} = \frac{\Delta P \cdot 4}{}$$	$\dot{V}$ = flow, πP = driving pressure 8 = constant, r = radius of airway π = pi	μ = viscosity of gas L = length of airway

Equation	Comments	Significance
Reynold's Number $Rn = \dfrac{v \times D \times d}{\mu}$	Rn = Reynold's # v = velocity of fluid D = density of fluid	d = diameter of tube μ = viscosity of fluid Rn < 2000 = laminar flow Rn > 2000 = turbulent
Temperature Conversion	$F = (C° \times 9/5) + 32°$ $C° = (F° - 32) \times 5/9$	See Appendix $K° = C° + 273$
Tobacco Use (Pack Years)	# Packs Smoked per Day x # Yrs Smkd	- There are usually 20 cigarettes/pk

10

Continued on Next Page

CONTENTS

PROCEDURES

Continued on Next Page

PROCEDURES

PROCEDURES

AEROSOL THERAPY

Types of Aerosol Therapy	**Bland Aerosol Delivery** (see AARC CPG, Next Page)
	Medicated Aerosol Delivery (See Also Chapter 12)

Hazards of Aerosol Therapy

- Adverse reaction to medication
- Airway obstruction (swollen mucus)
- Airway thermal injury
- Caregiver exposure to airborne contagion
- Bronchospasm
- Drug reconcentration
- Infection
- Overhydration (hypernatremia)
- Overmobilization of secretions
- Systemic effects

Bland Aerosol Administration[1, 2]

Indications

A bypassed upper airway (heated bland aerosol, MMAD 2-10 µ) [3]

Mobilization of secretions

Sputum induction (hypo or hypertonic saline, MMAD 1-5µ)

Upper airway edema – (cool bland aerosol, MMAD ≥ 5µ):
  Laryngotracheobronchitis
  Subglottic edema
  Post extubation edema
  Post-op management

Assessment of Need

One or more of stridor, croupy cough, hoarseness following extubation, Hx of upper airway irritation with ↑ WOB, LTB or croup, bypassed airway, or patient discomfort.

Hazards/Complications

Bronchoconstriction or wheezing: artificial airway or hyperton. sputum induction in COPD, asthma, CF, other)

Caregiver exposure to airborne contagion

Edema of airway wall or assoc. with ↓C + ↑Raw

Infection

Overhydration

Patient discomfort

Contraindications

Bronchoconstriction

History of airway hyper-responsiveness

Monitoring

Patient:

Respiratory – rate, pattern, mechanics, accessory muscle use, BS.

CV – rate, rhythm, BP

Response – pain, dyspnea, discomfort, restlessness.

Sputum – quantity, color, consistency, odor

Skin color

Pulse oximetry (if hypoxemia suspected)

Equipment – Spirometry if concern of adverse reaction.

Frequency

Post extubation – 4-8 hrs

Subglottic edema – until edema subsides

Bypassed upper airway – as long as bypassed

Sputum induction – prn

Clinical Goals

Water, hypo or isotonic saline:
↓ dyspnea, stridor, or WOB
Improved ABGs, O2 Sat, or VS

Hypertonic saline: sputum sample

1) Bland aerosol therapy is the administration of sterile water, hypotonic, isotonic or hypertonic saline with or without oxygen.
2) Adapted from the AARC Clinical Practice Guideline: Bland Aerosol Administration, 2003 Revision and Update, *Respiratory Care*, Vol. 48, #5, 2003.
3) Not as effective as heated water nebulizers or HME.

Aerosol Delivery Devices

Type	Use	Comments
Small Volume Nebulizer (SVN) *Also called handheld, mini-neb, mainstream, sidestream, slipstream, or in-line*	Used to deliver intermittent aerosolized medications Short-term use only Usually 2-5 mL of solution Optimal gas flow rates 6-8 L/min Average particle size 1-5 μm dia	Can be used with a mouthpiece, face mask, trach-collar, T-piece, or ventilator circuit, with normal breathing pattern and with all patients Need electrical, battery, or gas source to power Requires drug preparation Units can be either pneumatic or ultrasonic Use air, not oxygen, for patients on a hypoxic drive. Patient should take periodic deep breaths
Large Volume Nebulizer (LVN) (jet)	Used for continuous oxygen +/or aerosol therapy (heated or cool). Variable particle size 1-2 mL/min output	Can be used with a face mask, trach-collar, or T-piece. Condensation collects in tubing Correct solution level must be maintained ↑risk of nosocomial infection See air entrainment neb for air/O2 ratios, total V̇ Used primarily for patients with tracheostomies.
Ultrasonic (USN)	Used to mobilize thick secretions in the lower airways 90% of particles are 1-5 μm dia Usually only intermittent, but may be continuous therapy. 1-6 mL/min output	Drug preparation required Heat generated by USN may affect bronchodilators May precipitate bronchospasm, overmobilization of secretions, or overhydration. Not all drugs (e.g., Budesonide and Dornase) are compatible with ultrasonic nebulizers. Provides 100% humidity (continuous)

Type	Use	Comments
Metered Dose Inhaler (MDI)	Intermittent delivery of aerosolized medications. Particle size 3-6 μm	First method of choice. Small, easily cleaned Efficacy is design and technique dependent Inexpensive, convenient, portable, and no drug prep required Inspiratory flow rates should be ≤ 30 LPM May be used in-line with ventilators Patient self-administered, hence may not be appropriate for pediatric or geriatric patients. Requires hand-breath coordination, synchronization with inspiration, and a 4-10 sec. breath hold. Spacer or holding chamber is recommended, esp. with children.
Dry Powder Inhaler (DPI)	Intermittent delivery of a powdered medication. Particle size 1-2 μm	Breath actuated and patient self-administered Breath holding not required High humidity may affect some drugs. Many drugs unavailable in DPI form Not recommended for patients < 6 yrs or with acute broncho-spasm Some units require high flow rates (> 40 Lpm), hence may not be appropriate for pediatric or geriatric patients.
Small Particle Aerosol Generator (SPAG)	Delivery of aerosolized ribavirin.	Specific for ribavirin Caregiver precautions required

10-7

Device Selection

- ACCP and ACAAI evidence-based guidelines indicate that all aerosolized delivery systems are equally effective when used properly (Chest Jan, 2005).
- Selection should be based on drug availability, patient's abilities (cognitive, physical, learning, etc), patient preference, convenience, and cost.
- Selection of a specific device should be based on its ability to produce particles with a mass median aerodynamic diameter (MMAD) of 1-3 microns.

Overview

- CDC recommends that nebulizers be filled with sterile fluids (not tap or distilled H_2O), and be changed or replaced q 24 hrs.
- Cost, convenience, and the ease-of-use can affect compliance.
- Patient assessment before, during, and after therapy should include BS, breathing pattern, heart rate, overall appearance, and peak flow for patients with reactive airways.
- The efficacy of inhaled drugs can be affected by the device, the inhalation technique, severity of disease, and patient age.
- Unit dose (vs. multidose bottled) medications should be used.

Nebulizers

- Heated nebs require sterile solution and sterile immersion heaters, if used. Heaters must be monitored for proper funct.
- Nebulizers should be cleaned and changed periodically according to manufacturer recommendations.
- SVNs should be shaken, rinsed with either sterile or distilled water (not tap water), and left to air dry after each use. Drying may be enhanced by gas flow through the device after rinsing.

Newer types of nebulizers that are being studied or recently introduced into clinical practice include:

- Improvements in jet-nebulization (breath-actuated nebulizers)
- Vibrating mesh (porous membrane vibrating at ultrasonic frequencies)
- Pressurized liquids through a nozzle

These newer types of devices use less medication, are more efficient in aerosol delivery, and have little or no deadspace volume.

- **Counting**: Patients should be instructed to keep a tally of actuations used (including "wasted ones"), NOT by placing in a bowl of water.
- MDIs with a holding chamber or spacer reduces the need for patient coordination and improves particle deposition.
- MDI mouthpieces should be washed with mild soap and water every few days.
- Patient instruction and proper usage determines optimal delivery, and periodic assessment of proper technique is important.

MDI Technique
(see Pharmacology Chapter for device-specific information)

Without Accessory Device	With Accessory Device	
1. Assemble MDI, warm to body temperature		
2. Inspect mouthpiece for foreign matter		
3. Shake canister vigorously 3-4 shakes		
4. If > 24 hrs since last use, deliver one puff into the air (2-4 puffs if first use)	4a. Attach accessory device (spacer/holding chamber)	
5. Hold MDI upright and sit upright	b. Place mouthpiece or mask into accessory device	
6. Place mouthpiece 4 cm from open mouth (or between sealed lips for breath actuated device)	c. Place valve stem into canister holding orifice on accessory device	
7. Exhale normally		
8. Inspire slowly while depressing MDI canister at same time (inspiratory flow rate < 30 L/m or > 30 for breath actuated).	8a. If chamber is equipped with a reed device, prevent making a sound during inspiration.	
9. Continue inspiration until TLC	It is recommended that patients utilize a Spacer, but both techniques be taught for times when a pt doesn't have a spacer, or is noncompliant with spacer use.	
10. Hold breath 4-10 sec		
11. Wait 15-30 sec between puffs depending on medication (2 – 10 min for bronchodilators to enhance the effectiveness).		
12. Repeat as prescribed.		
13. Rinse mouth after use (esp. with corticosteroid use).		

Dry Powder Inhalers (DPI's)

Patient Instruction:
- Instruct patient to follow Doctor's orders precisely (# and freq. of treatments, medication dosage).
- Patient should be in sitting or high Fowler's position during therapy.
- Patients should be instructed in detecting any possible adverse reactions (see Pharmacology Chapter).
- Many times, Dry Powders do not have taste or texture - pt should be instructed that with proper technique, medication has been delivered despite no sensation to verify that.
- Patients should be instructed to cough, expectorate, or suction as needed.

Clinicians Should:
- Be familiar with the device and practiced with a placebo prior to instructing patients.
- Demonstrate assembly and correct use of device to patients.
- Per device specifications, clinician should verify pt's ability to use device - include inspiratory ability, as well as ability to coordinate/actuate.
- Provide written instructions on how to use the device and a written plan for use.
- Observe patient practice use of the device.

DPI Technique:

1. Assemble DPI and inspect mouthpiece for foreign matter
2. Load the medication (see device instructions)
3. Exhale normally (away from device)
4. Instruct pt to place mouthpiece in mouth, with lips sealed tightly, and inspire per manufacturer recommendations (some devices require short, quick inspiration while others require gradual inspiration)
5. Generally, inspiratory flow rate should be > 60 LPM
6. Hold breath 4-10 seconds
7. Repeat as prescribed
8. Rinse mouth after use (esp. with corticosteroid use).

Effective aerosol therapy requires the correct matching of appropriate device with the patient's ability to use it properly.

Selected Resources:

Respiratory Therapists	• A Guide to Aerosol Delivery Devices for Respiratory Therapists; Gardenhire, Ari, Hess, and Meyers; AARC (3rd Edition)
Health Care Professionals	• Guide to Aerosol Delivery Devices: For Physicians, Nurses, Pharmacists, and Other Health Care Professionals; Elliot and Dunne; AARC (2nd Edition, 2013)
Patients	• A Patient's Guide to Aerosol Drug Delivery; Gregory, Elliott, and, Dunne; AARC (1st Edition, 2013). aarc.org

Recommended particle sizes:

1-5 μ	sputum induction
2-5 μ	pharmacologically active aerosols
2-10 μ	bypassed upper airway
> 5 μ	upper airway administration

MMAD = mass medium aerodynamic diameter (μ)

It is important to again remember that MMAD can be affected by improper patient technique, resulting in inertial impaction, and ultimately less therapeutic deposition.

Selection of a Device for Delivery of Aerosol to the Lung Parenchyma[1]

Indication
The need to deliver a topical medication (in aerosol form) that has its site of action in the lung parenchyma or is intended for systemic absorption.

Contraindications
None, medication contraindications may exist.

Hazards/Complications
Malfunction of device, improper technique, medication complications, nebulizer design and characteristics of the medication may affect ventilator function and medication deposition, aerosols may cause bronchospasm or irritation of the airway, exposure to medications and patient-generated droplet nuclei may be hazardous to clinicians

Limitations
Efficacy of device is design and technique dependent, a relatively small fraction of nebulizer output deposits in the lung parenchyma (may be affected by MV, artificial airways, reduced airway caliber (eg, infants and pediatrics)

severity of obstruction, hydrophilic formulations, failure of patient to comply with procedure.

Assessment of Need
Availability of drug, formulation and equipment; superiority of any one method not established; cost, convenience, effectiveness, and patient tolerance of procedure should be considered; consider augmenting with MV when spontaneous ventilation is inadequate.

Assessment of Outcome/ Monitoring
Proper technique, compliance, response of patient, a positive clinical outcome.

Infection Control
Universal precautions, nebulizers should not be used between patients without disinfection, nebulizers should be changed or sterilized at conclusion of dose admin or every 24 hours; at 24-hour intervals with continuous admin; when visibly soiled.

CONTINUED ON NEXT PAGE

PROCEDURES

Selection of an Aerosol Delivery Device[1]
continued

Infection Control, cont. Nebulizers should not be rinsed with tap water between tx, but may be rinsed with sterile water. CDC recommends sterile water rinsing and air drying. All medications should be handled aseptically.	

1) Adapted from AARC Clinical Practice Guideline: Selection of a Device for Delivery of Aerosol to the Lung Parenchyma, *Respiratory Care*, Volume 41, 1996.

PROCEDURES

Notes *(this is a good place to keep your hospital-specific policies, procedures, and protocols related to aerosol delivery:*

Artificial Airways

Types and Indications

Type	Notes	Ventilation	Obstruction	Protection	Secretion
		Indications			
Oro-pharyngeal	Use only in unconscious patients with no cough or gag	X	X		X
Naso-pharyngeal	Useful in pts with (or at risk for developing) airway obstruction (particularly clenched jaw) May be better tolerated than oral airway in pts not deeply unconscious. Caution in pts with severe cranial facial injury		X		X
Endotracheal	Sizes vary - generally larger tubes offer less airway resistance, but should not be so large as to cause damage to vocal cords. See Below for further details.	X	X	X	X
Tracheostomy	Primarily used when Endotracheal Intubation not possible (or contraindicated), or with longer-term mechanical ventilation efforts	X	X	X	X

PROCEDURES

Endotracheal Tubes (ET Tubes)

Types:
- Regular (with Murphy Eye), usually slightly curved, pliable
- Subglottic tubes (allow for sx above the cuff)
- Anti-Aspiration Designs (microcuff, silver-coated, etc.)

Typical Sizing

	ET Tube I.D.(mm)	Avg Depth	Blade	Mask	Sx Catheter (Fr)
Adult Male	6.5-9.5	21-23	3-4	4	16
Adult Female	6.0-8.5	19-21	3	4	14

Tracheostomy Tubes (Trachs)

Types:

Characteristics	Typical Variations Available
Material	Metal (Jackson) Plastic (Shiley, Portex, Bivona, etc.)
Presence of Cuff	Cuffed or Uncuffed
Type of Cuff	Air, Fluid, or Foam Filled
Shape	Normal versus Speciality (Distal, Proximal, Custom)
Fenestrations	Fenestrated or Unfenestrated
Inner Cannula	None or Removable (Nondisposable, Disposable)
Adjuncts	Speaking Valves (see next page)
Sizes	Vary, Adult usually 4-9

A Speaking Valve is a one-way valve (pt can inhale via trach, but then must exhale through upper airway). Cuffed trachs MUST HAVE THE CUFF FULLY DEFLATED when speaking valve is in place.

Indications for Tracheostomy Placement

- Patients unable to protect their airways
- Excessive secretions
- Failure of noninvasive methods of cough assist
- Swallowing or cough impairment with chronic aspiration
- Patients requiring invasive ventilation > 21 days
- Contraindications to, failed, or cannot tolerate NPPV
- Need to reduce anatomical deadspace for improved oxygenation and/or ventilation

Speaking Valves

Common Brands	• Passy Muir Valve (PMV) • Shiley • Montogomery
Purposes	• Pt Communication • Facilitates swallowing (eating/drinking) • Pt may retain Instrinsic PEEP • Better Secretion Management (cough secretions to upper airway)
Procedure	• **DEFLATE TRACH CUFF**
	• Attach speaking valve to trach • If needed, increase VT on Vent-Dependent pts (leak has been created) • On initial placement, monitor for tolerance: HR, RR, SpO$_2$, WOB, Dyspnea • If indicated, attach O$_2$ to valve
Problems	• Air-trapping • Fatigue • Mucus can occlude one-way valve • Tolerance of Valve

Tracheostomy Troubleshooting Guide

Complication	Possible Causes	Possible Actions
Balloon won't stay inflated	Cuff patent?	Consider Trach Change
Bleeding	Amount in relation to when trach placed/ changed last	Immediately Consult MD
Chest Pain	R/O Cardiac misplaced Trach Occluded Trach Resp Failure	Request EKG Verify Placement of Trach
Crackling and/ or Edema around stoma	Trach in tissue (sub-q. air)	Verify Placement* Consider Trach Change (notify MD per policy)
High Cuff Pressures Should be < 30 mmHg	Incorrect Size?	Consider Trach Change if larger trach due to risk of tracheomalacia over time
Difficulty passing Sx Catheter	Sx Catheter too large? Misplaced Trach? Occluded Trach?	**Consider Lavage. If still un- able to pass sx, and/or pt distress, immed. pull trach** If occluded from dried mucus, ensure adequate humidity and sx'ing
Drying of Tracheal Mucosa	Lack of Humidity?	Consider adding Heated (or Cool) Humidity
Excessive Secre- tions, Change in Secretions	Infection? Lack of Humidity?	Consider Culturing Add Humidity Bronchial Hygiene
Redness of Skin around Tube, Drainage	Infection (may be SOB, febrile)	Consider Culturing Wound Care consult?
Granulation Tissue (immature blood vessels)	Complication of Trach in place for extend. period May Bleed Easily	Consider regular trach changes (1-2 weeks)
Excessive Cough- ing, Gagging, SOB, Choking	Excessive Secretions Tolerance	Bronchial Hygiene Instill Lidocaine (cautious!) Mech Ventilation?

Replacing a Trach Tube*
(see Important Trach Change Considerations, Next Page)

Inner Cannula

1. Explain procedure to patient
2. Position patient supine or slightly elevated
3. Perform hand hygiene, apply gloves. Consider face shield/mask
4. Have patient take a deep breath in
5. Insert inner cannula gently and lock in place

Replacing Trach

1. Explain procedure to patient
2. Position patient supine or slightly elevated
3. Perform hand hygiene, apply gloves. Consider face shield/mask
4. Clean area (use sterile water), then dry
5. Remove inner cannula of new tube (if present), insert obturator. Check new cuff for leaks (if present).
6. Lubricate outside of tube with water-soluble lubricant
7. Stand on side of pt to avoid exposure to body fluids from trach
8. Oxygenate (if needed), suction inserted trach and upper airway, re-oxygenate
9. Remove holder/tie, have patient take a deep breath (or give deep breath with resuscitation bag), <u>deflate cuff</u>, then remove old trach tube gently
10. Quickly, but gently, insert new tube (sideways, then gently downward) (do not force), hold tube in place and immediately remove obturator
11. Insert inner cannula and lock in place (if present), inflate cuff, if present
12. **Verify placement (ETCO$_2$, pass suction catheter, auscultate, feel for air flow). Remove tube if cannot be placed properly or airflow is inadequate; ventilate as needed and attempt to reinsert tube.**
13. Hold tube in place until urge to cough subsides
14. Secure trach holder/ties (leave one finger width loose)
15. Suction and oxygenate if needed. Reauscultate/assess
16. Perform hand hygiene and document procedure

* The frequency of tube change depends on airway size, presence of cough, secretion volume and color, malfunction, or grossly dirty or contaminated.

Commonly, adult, cuffed tubes, q 4-8 weeks; uncuffed tubes, q 6 months. Children typically require more frequent changes, due to growth changes.

PROCEDURES

Tracheostomy Tube Care

1. Perform hand hygiene, put gloves on. Consider face shield/mask
2. Open all packages
3. Suction trach tube before removing
4. Remove inner cannula by unlocking/gently pulling outward or re-move single tube or outer cannula by cutting ties, holding tube in place with finger, deflate cuff, pull gently outward and downward.
5. Soak tube in cleaning solution for indicated time
6. Clean skin/stoma with cotton dipped in sol. + pat dry with gauze.
7. Brush inside of tube with cleaning solution
8. Rinse tube thoroughly with distilled water
9. Pat dry with clean gauze and replace

Considerations for Trach Changes

Variable	Considerations
Equipment	Always have a BVM at the ready, connected to O_2 with appropriate flow running. Intubation equip. should be easily accessible.
People at Bedside	Per policy, with minimum of one person changing trach and one other qualified medical professional who can assist with airway management
Age of Trach	Fresh tracheostomies (< 1 week old) should be changed only if emergent, and by MD. Risk of loss of patent airway if pulled. Intubation equipment should be present.
Anatomical	**Extreme Caution Should be Used in:** • Obese Patients • Abnormal neck anatomy • Any trach placed for patency (versus ventilation/oxygenation)
Size	Downsizing is generally easier than replacing same size, and extreme caution in upsizing.
Verification	Always verify correct placement following a trach change. Use Auscultation, ETCO2, Chest Rise, Return Volumes if on Vent, SpO2, WOB, ability to pass sx catheter and/or able to "bag" patient effectively

PROCEDURES

- Inspect Stoma site daily for secretions, signs of infection/ inflammation (redness), and encrustation (granuloma formation). Document/report all skin breakdown per policy.
- Clean stoma at least daily (more freq if breakdown) with cotton-tipped applicator and water or 1:1 hydrogen peroxide and water or saline solution. Apply Betadine/Polyspirin PRN.
- Change dressing at least once a day
- Trach ties (both velcro and cloth) should be changed as needed. With the flange of the trach tube secured, remove dirty tie and replace with a new, properly sized one, making sure the tie is secure, but not too tight. One finger should fit beneath tie.

Capping and Decannulation *(normal progression)*

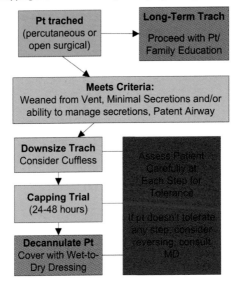

Choosing Humidity Therapy for Patients with Tracheostomies

	Heated Humidifier	Nebulizer	HME-HCH
Efficacy	**Good:** Efficient, temperature control preferred for long term trach ventil.	**Fair:** May be too cool, heaters not very practical, may deliver too much water	**Fair:** Not for thick, copious secretions, marginal humidity, can't use with speaking valves May be used for periods <12 hrs if min secretions
Safety	**Fair:** May cause burns, electrical hazard, inadvertent lavage from condensation	**Fair:** Water droplets may cause bronchospasm - del. excess H2O	**Fair:** No power or condensation hazards, may occlude with secretions, ↑Raw
Cost	Expensive	Fair	Fair
Convenience	**Poor:** Complex (with heated wire), condensation (w/o heated wire), water refill > 8 hr	**Fair:** Simple, water refill < 8 hr	**Good:** Simple, no additional equipment needed

SEE ALSO: Humidity Therapy, this chapter

SEE ALSO: Humidity Therapy, this chapter

Intubation Procedure

Prepare all Equipment, and Fully Assess the Patient prior to intubating:

- Bag and Valve Mask Ventilation (BVM) connected to O2 (12-15 L)
- Laryngoscope (check bulb)
- Blades (Miller or MacIntosh)
- Endotracheal Tube (several sizes), check cuff
  Use new Endotracheal Tube on each Intubation attempt
- 10 cc Syringe
- Stylet (flexible or rigid, depending on intubation apparatus)
- ETCO2 detector, capnography, EDD, etc. for verifying placement

IMPORTANT CONSIDERATIONS:

- Have all possible equipment at bedside to anticipate difficulties (fiberoptic equipment, bronchoscope, etc.)
- Cautious Rapid Sequence Intubation (RSI) in pts who are obese, who are known difficult intubations, etc.
- Pulse Oximetry, Blood Pressure, and EKG must be monitored during intubation. Interrupt attempt if oxygenation/ventilation is needed
- Only direct visualization is completely reliable. Use all possible verification methods. IF IN DOUBT, PULL IT OUT
- Remove tube at once if gurgling in stomach, and no chest expansion

Insertion Distance: Male (21-23 cm); Female (19-21 cm)

Successful Intubation Checklist:

	Lungs: equal + bilateral breath sounds, Chest Expans.
	Abdomen: ↓ sounds in abdom, No + abdom. distention
	Warm air exhaled from ET Tube
	+ ETCO$_2$* (Yellow is YES, Purple is PROBLEM)
	Condensate inside of ET Tube
	Improved patient color/SpO$_2$
	Visualization with bronchocope (if at bedside)
	CXR Verification
	Esophageal Detector Device (EDD)*

*See further ETCO$_2$ and EDD considerations on following page.

PROCEDURES

End-tidal CO₂ Detector ($P_{ET}CO_2$) for Verification

CO₂ Detected	
Tube likely in trachea	May rarely detect CO_2 if tube in esophagus and lg amts of carbonated fluid ingested prior to. This will dissipate after a few ventilations.
CO₂ Not Detected	
Tube is in Esophagus	• Absent Chest Rise • Absent Breath Sounds • Stomach gurgling and distension

Tube is in Trachea
 	
Verify with several other methods
	Decreased CO₂ IN Lungs:
	  • Poor blood flow to lungs
	  • Cardiac Arrest
	  • Pulmonary Embolus
	  • IV Bolus of Epinephrine
	
	Decreased CO₂ FROM Lungs:
	  • Airway Obstruct (Status Asthm., etc.)
	  • Pulmonary Edema
	  • Mucus Plugging

Unclear Where Tube Is	Detector Contaminated with gastric contents or acidic drug
ETCO₂ device applied incorrectly, Time	Many disposable devices require "activation" (such as by pulling of paper tab), and may req. a few ventilations to change color

Esophageal Detector Device for Verification

Syringe-Type plunger is attached to ET Tube.	
Able to Pull Back on Plunger	ET Tube likely in trachea (rigid structure of trachea allows for air passage)
Unable to Pull Back on Plunger	ET Tube likely in esophagus (floppy structure of esophagus collapses over end of ET tube)
Caution: May be misleading in morbid obesity, late pregnancy, status asthmaticus, or with copious secretions. Use in Children only if > 20 kg with perfusing rhythm.	

Management of Airway Emergencies[1]

Indications

Conditions requiring general airway management: airway compromise, protection, respiratory failure.

Conditions requiring emergency tracheal intubation, surgical placement or alternative techniques (see the AARC guideline for a list of numerous specific conditions).

Contraindications

Patient's documented desire not to be resuscitated.

Monitoring

Patient:

Clinical signs – airway obstruction (blood, foreign objects, secretions, vomitus), BS, chest movement, epigastric sounds, LOC, nasal flaring, retractions, skin color, upper airway sounds (snoring, stridor), ventilation ease.

Physiologic variables – ABG, pulse ox., CXR, $PeCO_2$, HR, rhythm, f, V_T, Paw.

Tube positioned in trachea:

Confirmed by – chest x-ray, endoscopic visualization, exhaled CO_2

Suggested by – BS (bilateral), chest movement (symmetrical), condensate upon exhalation, epigastrium (absence of ventilation sounds), esophageal detector devices, visualization of passage through vocal cords.

Precautions/Hazards/Complications

Emergency Ventilation:

barotrauma, gastric insufflation/rupture, hypo/hyper ventilation, hypotension, O_2 delivery (inadequate), unstable cervical spine, upper airway obstruction, ventilation (prolonged interruption), vomiting, aspiration.

Trans-Laryngeal intubation, Cricothyroidotomy:

Aspiration, bronchospasm, laryngospasm, bradycardia, tachycardia, dysrhythmia, hypo/hypertension,

ET tube problems –
Cuff herniation, perforation, extubation (inadvertent), pilot tube valve incompetence, size inappropriate, tube kinking, occlusion.

Failure to establish patient airway, intubate the trachea

Intubation of bronchi, esophagus

Pneumonia

Trauma – airway, cervical spine, dental, esophagus, eye, nasal, needle cricothyroidotomy (bleeding, esophageal perforation, subcutaneous emphysema), vocal cords.

Ulceration, stenosis, malacia

1) Adapted from the AARC Clinical Practice Guidelines: Management of Airway Emergencies, *Respiratory Care*, Volume 40, #7, 1995.

PROCEDURES

Bag and Valve Mask Ventilation (BVM)

Variable	Considerations	
Rates	**Most Pts**	10-12 breaths/min (every 5-6 sec) with 1 sec inspir.
	COPD ↑ **Raw Hypovol.**	6-8 breaths/min (every 7-10 sec) with 1 sec inspir. - avoids Auto-PEEP -
	CPR	8-10 breaths/min - allows venous return -
Volumes	**Estimated (deliver enough for visible chest rise):**	
	Adult	500-600 mL (6-7 mL/kg) 1 L Adult Bag: 1/2 - 2/3 vol 2 L Adult Bag: 1/3 vol
	Infant/ Child	Visible Chest Rise Bag size should be > 450-500 mL
Gas Source	Run at 15+ L/min of Oxygen. Verify flow is from Oxygen outlet/tank, verify tubing is connected	
Personnel	Most effective with 2 Rescuers - 1 opens airway/seals mask, 2nd squeezes bag while both observe chest rise	
Cautions	**Avoid Hyperinflation**	
	Giving > 12 breaths/min (> every 5 sec) may ↑ PIT, ↓venous return, ↓CO, and ↓ coronary and cerebral perfusion.	
	Gastric inflation	
	Giving large or forceful breaths may cause regurgitation, aspiration, elevated diaphragm, ↓ lung movement, and ↓ CL.	
	Patient Vomits	
	Turn to side, wipe/sx out mouth, return to Supine	
Inadequate Face/Mask Ventilation	• Absent or ↓: bs, chest movement, expired CO_2 • ↓ SpO_2, Cyanosis • Excessive gas leak • Gastric air entry/dilatation • Hemodyn. changes (↑HR, ↑ BP, arrhythmias)	

- A natural (strong) cough is the best method of clearing secretions. Manually assisted coughing or mechanical cough assist (see Lung Expansion Therapy, this Chapter) may reduce the need for suctioning.
- Routine and frequent suctioning is not recommended. Suction catheters traumatize the airway mucosa potentially increasing secretion production, may cause hypoxemia and/or cardiac arrhythmias, possible atelectasis, as well as the risk of infection.
- When suctioning is necessary, perform as gently as possible, keeping the catheter within the tube, if possible.
- If suctioning beyond the tube tip is necessary, the catheter should be advanced gently and suction applied only during catheter withdrawal, with suction being applied for no more than 15 sec.
- Use the lowest suction pressure possible to obtain the desired result. If suction catheter becomes clogged, quickly clear out obstruction, do not increase suction.

Indications/Need

Evidence of Secretions	• Visible secretions in tube • Audible course, wet, +/or ↓ BS • Palpation of wet, course vibrations through chest wall

Alterations in Patient or Ventilation	• Patient:
	  ↑ agitation, irritability, restless
	• Ventilator: ↑ Raw
	  VV: ↑ PIP and ↑ high pressure alarms
	  PV: ↓ VT

Alterations in Vital Signs	• Change in respiratory pattern:
	  ↑ WOB, tachypnea, retractions
	• Change in cardiac pattern:
	  ↑ or ↓ HR

Alterations in O_2 and Ventilation	• ↓ SpO2 (< 90%) • Skin color changes – pale, dusky, or cyanotic • Changes in ABGs - ↑ PaCO2, ↓ PaO2, respiratory acidosis

PROCEDURES

Suction Pressures/Catheter Sizes

Suction Pressures	Suction Catheter Size
Adult -100 to -150* mm Hg Child -80 to -100 mm Hg Infant -60 to -80 mm Hg *some sources = -120 mmHg	ET tube size (ID) x 2, then use next smaller size suction catheter E.g.; 6.0 x 2 = 12, use 10 FR

Suctioning Procedure

1. Assess indications/need as above
2. Set up and test suction pressure (never use "Max")
3. Explain procedure to patient ("this will make you cough")
4. Position patient: (commonly, unless contraindicated)
   Nasaotracheal and pharyngeal suctioning – Semi-Fowler's position with neck hyperextended
   Endotracheal and tracheostomy – supine
5. Wash and glove both hands – use sterile technique
6. Pre-oxygenate with 100% O₂ for 30 sec
7. Note RR, HR, and SpO₂, and monitor throughout procedure
8. Insert catheter as far as possible (until you feel resistance, or until patient begins to cough), then withdraw a few cm. (For ET or trach tubes, advance to just past ET tube tip [shallow sx] or until meet resistance at carina and then withdraw 1 cm [deep sx])
9. Apply suction while withdrawing and rotating the catheter (~ 10-15 sec). Do not move catheter up and down. Stop and remove immediately if untoward patient response.
10. Allow patient to rest and reoxygenate for 1 minute
11. Clean secretions from catheter by suctioning sterile water
12. Monitor patient (vital signs and response)
13. Repeat steps 6-11 as needed (usually no more than 2-3 passes with catheter)
14. Return any continuous O₂ to pre-suction settings

NOTES for FOLLOWING PAGE (Nasotracheal Suctioning CPG):
1) The insertion of a suction catheter through the nasal passage and pharynx into the trachea (without a tracheal tube or tracheostomy) to remove material from the trachea and nasopharynx that cannot be removed by the patient's spontaneous cough.
2) Adapted from the AARC Clinical Practice Guideline: Nasotracheal Suctioning, *Respiratory Care*, Volume 37, #8, 1992 and 2004 update.

Nasotracheal Suctioning[1,2]
(AARC Expert Panel Reference-Based Guideline)

Indications
Patient's cough unable to clear secretions or foreign material in the large central airways.
Evidenced by:
  Audible or visible secretions in airway
  Chest x-ray (retained secretions → atelectasis or consolidation)
  Coarse, gurgling BS or ↓ BS
  Hypoxemia or hypercarbia
  Suspected aspiration
  Tactile fremitus
  ↑WOB
To stimulate cough or for un-relieved coughing
To obtain sputum sample

Contraindications
Absolute: Croup or epiglottis
Relative: Acute facial, head or neck injury, bronchospasm, coagulopathy or bleeding disorder, high gastric surgery, irritable airway, laryngospasm, MI, nasal bleeding, occluded nasal passages, tracheal surgery, URI.

Pressures
Adult   -100 to -150 mm Hg
Child   -100 to -120 mm Hg
Infant   -80 to -100 mm Hg
Neonate -60 to -80 mm Hg

Suction time should be < 15 sec.

Frequency
Only when indicated and other measures have failed.

Monitoring
(before, during, and after)
BS, cough, CV parameters (HR, BP, EKG), ICP, laryngospasm, oxygen saturation, RR, pattern, SpO2, skin color, sputum (color, volume, consistency, odor), subjective response (pain), trauma, bleeding.

Hazards/Complications
Atelectasis, bronchospasm, CV changes (↓ HR,↑↓BP, arrhythmia, arrest), gagging, vomiting, hypoxia, hypoxemia,↑ ICP (IVH, cerebral edema), laryngospasm, mechanical trauma (bleeding, irritation, laceration, perforation, tracheitis), misdirection of catheter, nosocomial infection, pain, pneumo-thorax, respiratory arrest, uncontrolled coughing.

Assessment of Outcome
Improved BS, improved ABGs or SpO2, secretions removed, ↓WOB (↓RR or dyspnea)

See footnotes for this CPG on PREVIOUS PAGE

Notes:

Airway Clearance Techniques

Variable	Considerations
Indications	**Prevent Secretion Retention** Acute respiratory failure; Atelectasis; Immobile patients; Lung disease (COPD, etc.); Neuromuscular disorders; Post Op? **Remove Copious Secretions** Allergens/irritants; Asthma; Bronchiectasis; Bronchitis; Cystic fibrosis; Infection **Copious Secretions = 25-30 mL/day (1oz/shot glass)**
Signs & Symptoms	**Symptoms** ↑ Chest congestion; ↑ Cough (or ineffective); ↑ SOB or WOB; ↑ Wheezing; ↑ or ↓ Sputum product **Signs** BS – abnormal, audible or ↓; ↑ RR, ↑ HR; ↑ Respiratory tract infections and fever; ↓ SpO2 or worsening ABG's; ↓ Expiratory flow rates; Secretions - ↓ or ↑, thick, or discolored; Chest X-ray changes **Note**: The effectiveness of bronchial hygiene therapy is commonly determined by improvement of the above signs & symptoms
Factors Affecting Secretion Clearance	**Impaired Mucocilliary Transport** Analgesics; Anesthetics; Cigarette smoking; Cuffed ET or trach tube ; Dehydration (dry gases > 4 L/m, bypass of upper airway); Electrolyte imbalance; Hypoxia or hypercapnia; Loss of cilia (COPD, infection); Pollutants **Impaired Cough Force** Abdominal restriction, surgery, pain; Air trapping (emphysema); Airway collapse, constriction, inflammation, obstruction (allergens, asthma, CF, COPD, infection, irritants, tumors); Artificial airway; CNS depression; Drugs (analgesics/ narcotics); NM weakness, fatigue, paralysis, **Excessive or Thick Secretions** Allergens/irritants; Asthma; Bronchiectasis; Bronchitis; Cystic fibrosis; Infection

PROCEDURES

Selecting Bronchial Hygiene Therapies

Patient Concerns	Technique Factors
• Ability to self administer is an important factor • Disease type and severity • Fatigue or work required • Pt's age and ability to learn • Patient's pref. and goals	• Clinician skill in teaching the technique • Cost (direct and indirect) • Equipment required • Physician/caregiver goals • Therapy effectiveness

See Bronchial Hygiene Selection Algorithm (pg 10-56) and ACCP Recommendations (pg 10-57)

Make Choices Based Upon the above factors/concerns, but as with most therapies you should consider Least Intense options first, moving to more intense options as a therapy is not effective, or not appropriate for pt clinical condition / ability.

Suggested Order of Therapy Implementation

Least Intense (Self)	• Directed Cough *+ • Diaphragmatic Exercises *+ • Pursed Lip Breathing • Autogenic Drainage/ACBT
(Device)	• Acapella Device • Flutter Valve
Intense (Device + Time)	• Postural Drainage, Percuss. & Vibration*+ • The Vest (and others) *+ • In-Exsufflator (Cough Assist) * • Intrapulmonary Percussive Ventil. (IPV)*+ • Nasotracheal Suctioning (NTS)
Most Intense	• Therapeutic Bronchoscopy *+ • Intubation (Short-Term) • Tracheostomy (Longer-Term)

* Options for Patients with Non-Vented Patients w/ Artificial Airways
+ Options for Patients who are Mechanically Ventilated

Directed or Therapeutic Coughing

Indications	May assist in pts with limited cough ability, who are weak/deconditioned, but with adequate neurological function to follow/learn instructions	
Techniques	**Controlled Cough**	Three deep breaths, exhaling normally after the first two and then coughing firmly on the third.
	Double Cough	A deep breath followed by two coughs with the second cough more forceful.
	Three Coughs	A small breath and a fair cough, then a bigger breath and a harder cough, and finally a deep breath with a forceful cough.
	Pump Coughing	A deep breath followed by three short easy coughs, then three huffs.
	Huff Cough (Forced Expiratory Technique [FET])	A slow, deep breath (mid-lung) followed by a 1-3 sec hold, then a series of short, quick, forceful exhalations or "huffs" with the mouth and glottis kept open.
	Manually-Assisted Cough	A deep breath followed by a forceful exhalation, plus an assistant quickly and firmly pushing the abdomen (or lateral costal margins of chest) up against the diaphragm during exhalation. *
Contra-indications	Pregnant women, abdominal pathologies, (e.g., aortic aneurysm, hiatal hernia), and/or unconscious patient with unprotected airways. Lateral costal margin pressure is contraindicated with osteoporosis or flail chest. ACCP does not recommend for patients with airflow obstruction, like COPD.	

PROCEDURES

Directed Cough[1,2]

Indications
Atelectasis, post-op prophylaxis, secretion retention/removal, sputum sampling.

Contraindications
Relative: acute unstable head neck or spine injury; ↓coronary artery perfusion (acute MI), inability to control droplet nuclei transmission (TB), ↑ICP, intracranial aneurysm.

Manually assisted cough to epigastrum: abdominal aortic aneurysm, acute abdominal pathology, bleeding diathesis, hiatal hernia, ↑risk of regurgitation/aspiration, pregnancy, untreated pneumothorax.

Manually assisted cough to thorax: flail chest, osteoporosis.

Frequency
PRN, post-op prophylaxis (q 2-4 hrs while awake), during and at end of any bronchial hygiene, FET (as alternative for PDT) (tid, 4 times/day).

Hazards/Complications
Anorexia, vomiting, retching, barotrauma, bronchospasm, central line displacement, chest pain, cough paroxysms, ↓cerebral perfusion, ↓coronary artery perfusion, fatigue, gastroesophageal reflux, headache, incisional pain, evisceration, incontinence, muscle damage/discomfort, paresthesia/numbness, rib or cartilage fracture, vertebral artery dissection, visual disturbance.

Monitoring
Adverse neurologic signs, BS, cardiac arrhythmias, hemodynamic alterations, patient's subjective response (pain, dyspnea, discomfort), pulmonary mechanics (PEF, PEP, PIP, Raw, VC), sputum.

Clinical Goals
Improved: clinical status, subjective response
Sputum production
Stabilized pulmonary hygiene

1) A component of any bronchial hygiene therapy when spontaneous cough is inadequate. Includes forced expiratory technique (FET or huff cough) and manually assisted cough.
FET = one or two huffs (forced expiration) from mid to low lung volume with an open glottis (often with brisk abduction of the upper arms), followed by a period of diaphragmatic breathing and relaxation.
Manually assisted cough = external application of mechanical pressure to epigastric region or thoracic cage during forced exhalation.
2) Adapted from AARC Clinical Practice Guideline: Directed Cough, *Respiratory Care*, Vol. 38, #5, 1993.

Active Cycle of Breathing Techniques (ACBT)	
Technique	1. Gentle diaphragmatic breathing at normal VT with relaxation of upper chest and shoulders. 2. Four thoracic expansion exercisees (TEE) - deep inspirations and relaxed expiration 3. Repeat #1 4. Forced Expiration Technique (FET) consists of one or two huffs at appropriate lung volume, dependent on location of secretions, followed ALWAYS by breathing control #1 (e.g. one or two mid- to low-lung volume huffs, if secretions located in more peripheral airways, one or tow high lung volume huffs or cough, if secretions located in larger more central airways followed by #1. 5. Repeat cycle until chest is as clear as possible.
Note	• Avoid cough until secretions for expectoration in upper airways • Intersperse with #1 at any stage, if patient becomes breathless or wheezy

Autogenic Drainage	
Indications	Primarily used for Cystic Fibrosis, though may assist with others with thick secretions. Because of technique required, pt should be > 8 yrs old.
Techniques	• Requires several sessions to learn technique, but is then a self-directed (no equipment) therapy: • Instruct pt to sit or recline, with neck slightly extended. • Three Phases:

Phase 1 *(Unstick)*	• Inhale small lung volume with a 1-3 sec breath hold • Exhale actively, but not forcefully • Repeat 1-3 minutes until secretions mobilized and heard/ felt in larger middle sized airways (ie, crackles - coarse and loud)	
Phase 2 *(Collect)*	• Inhale medium lung volume with a 1-3 sec breath hold • Exhale actively, but not forcefully • Repeat 1-3 minutes until secretions mobilized and heard/ felt in largest proximal airways (ie crackles - coarser and louder)	
Phase 3 *(Evacuate)*	• Inhale, slow, deep breaths (large lung volumes), with a 1-3 sec breath hold • Exhale actively, more forcefully • Repeat until secretions expectorated with huff or controlled cough • Follow with #1. • Repeat cycle until chest is as clear as possible.	

Diaphragmatic Exercises

Indications	• Alleviate Dyspnea;Improve Oxygenation • Increase Ventilation; Reduce Post-Op Complications
Technique	• Have pt assume comfortable position (sitting supported, semi-fowlers, or supine with hip and knees flexed). • Explain purpose, goals, demonstrate desired result. • Place hand on pt's epigastric area, asking them to breathe slowly and comfortably; follow pt's breathing with hand. • Pursed-lip breathing (as described later in this chapter) is often performed with diaphragmatic breathing. • After several breathing cycles, as the pt completes an exhalation, apply a firm counter-pressure with the hand and ask the patient to inhale and to "fill my hand with air"; observe the expansion under your hand, then instruct pt to exhale normally. • Continue practicing, then have the patient place his or her own hand on their epigastric area and repeat the procedure. • Continue practicing until the pt can perform the exercise properly w/ no verbal cues or having hand on their epigastrium. • As an aid to teaching, the patient may place his other hand over the sternum and instruct the patient to keep that hand from moving up and down. • Advance teaching can be done by having the patient perform the exercise while sitting unsupported, standing, and walking.

PROCEDURES

Diaphragmatic Strengthening

Indications	Patients with less than normal diaphragmatic strength
Technique	• The application of progressively increasing manual resistance or weights applied over the epigastric area with the patient in the supine position. • The patient should perform several series of three to five slow sustained deep diaphragmatic breaths with interposed rest periods. • Proper starting weight or pressure should permit full epigastric rise for 15 minutes with no signs of accessory muscle contraction. • Additional weight is added as strength improves.
Note	Positioning the patient in a Trendelenburg position, using the force of abdominal contents to resist the diaphragm, can accomplish the same results. A 15° head down tilt results in approximately 10 lbs. of force against the diaphragm. (Caution when using head-down position, see pg 10-48).

Pursed-Lip Breathing

Indications	To improve ventilation and oxygenation in patients with air-trapping (Asthma, COPD, etc.)
Technique	• Instruct patient to inhale slowly through the nose • Patient is then told to exhale gently through pursed lips (as though whistling) without any use of abdominal muscles. One part of the breathing cycle should be for inspiration and two parts for exhalation (e.g., 2 sec for TI and 4 sec for TE). • If performed while walking; 2 steps as the patient breathes in and 4 steps as the patient breathes out. E must always be longer than I.

PROCEDURES

Chest Physiotherapy (CPT)

Indications	Particularly beneficial in Cystic Fibrosis, May benefit patients with thick, secretions (?)
Technique	• Perform at least 1 hr before or 2 hrs after meals. • Prescribed bronchodilator therapy should be given 15 min before therapy. • Ensure patient loosens any tight or binding clothing. • Drainage should begin with superior segments and progress downward. Lung Segment to be drained should be placed such that main bronchus is pointing ↓ (use of pillows/blankets may assist in positioning) • Maintain position for 3-20 min, depending on quantity and tenacity of secretions and patient tolerance. Limit total treatment time to 30-40 min. • Appply Percussion and Vibration (see next page) • Have patient cough q 5 min during each position and after therapy (use FET in head down positions). There will be less of a rise in ICP if pt is in upright position during cough.

Monitoring	• Watch for signs of patient intolerance and monitor heart rate, BP, and SpO_2 during tx,
	• Signs of respiratory compromise:
	    • ↓ diaphragm excusion in head-down position
	    • Airway obstruction from secretions/collapse
	• ALL THERAPY SHOULD BE ADJUSTED BASED UPON PT'S CLINICAL CONDITION / TOLERANCE

Clinical Notes	• Oxygen requirements may increase during CPT, but should decrease following. Positional changes will alter V/Q and may be either beneficial or detrimental to Oxygenation/Ventilation • **NOTE**: Owing to the potential detrimental side effects and recent evidence showing a beneficial effect of using modified positioning, head-down positioning is no longer recommended to be used with PD&P in neo/peds, by the CF Foundation and various CPG's in Australia, Canada, and Europe. • Controversy still remains about using the head down position in adults. Adults have the ability to voice discomfort and intolerance of a therapy.

PROCEDURES

Percussion and Vibration	
Indications	Particularly beneficial in Cystic Fibrosis, May benefit patients with thick, secretions
Technique	• Percussion is applied to various lung segments either manually (with cupped hands) or mechanically with a motorized percussor/vibrator type unit (electric or pneumatic). • Chest percussion or clapping and vibration are often used in conjunction with postural drainage. • Percussion or clapping is usually applied for several minutes or as tolerated by the patient. • The therapist should remove rings/jewelry on hands/wrist. • Percussion is followed by vibration on exhalation. • Vibration is applied to the chest area with hands tensing at 6-8 vibrations per second for 4-6 exhalations. • The procedure concludes with a deep cough (several techniques are described in this chapter) and expulsion of secretions. • Patients should be allowed to rest as each lung segment is drained and cleared. • Should not be performed on a bare chest, over heart, stomach, spine, kidneys, women's breasts, chest tubes, incisions, wounds, fractures.

Hospitalized Patients without Cystic Fibrosis

1. Chest physiotherapy is not recommended for the routine treatment of uncomplicated pneumonia.
2. Airway Clearance Techniques are not recommended for routine use in patients with COPD.
3. Airway Clearance Techniques may be considered in patients with COPD with symptomatic secretion retention, guided by patient preference, toleration, and effectiveness of therapy.
4. Airway Clearance Techniques are not recommended if the patient is able to mobilize secretions with cough, but instruction in effective cough technique (FET) may be useful.

Neuromuscular Disease, Respiratory Muscle Weakness, or Impaired Cough

1. Cough assist techniques should be used in patients with neuromusclar disease, particularly when peak cough flow is < 270 L/min.
2. CPT, PEP, IPV, and HFCWC is not recommended.

Postoperative

1. Incentive spirometry is not recommended for routine, prophylactic use in postoperative patients.
2. Early mobility and ambulation is recommended to reduce postop complications and promote airway clearance.
3. Airway Clearance Techniques are not recommended for routine postoperative care.

[1] Adapted from AARC Clinical Practice Guideline: Effectiveness of Nonpharmacologic Airway Clearance Therapies in Hospitalized Patients, Respiratory Care, Dec 2013, Vol 58, #12.

[2] Guidelines are appropriate for adult and pediatric populations

PROCEDURES

Effectivenesss of Pharmacologic Airway Clearance Therapies in Hospitalized Patients[1, 2]
AARC Clinical Practice Guideline Summary

Hospitalized Patients without Cystic Fibrosis

1. Recombinant human dornase alfa should not be used in patients with non-cystic fibrosis bronchiectasis.
2. Routine use of bronchodilators to aid in secretion clearance is not recommended.
3. Routine use of aersolized N-acetylcysteine to improve airway clearance is not recommended.

Neuromuscular Disease, Respiratory Muscle Weakness, or Impaired Cough

The use of aerosolized agents to change sputum physical properties or improve airway clearance is not recommended.

Postoperative

1. Mucolytics is not recommended for use in the treatment of atelectasis.
2. Routine administration of bronchodilators is not recommended.

[1]Adapted from AARC Clinical Practice Guideline: Effectiveness of Pharmacologic Airway Clearance Therapies in Hospitalized Patients, Respiratory Care, July 2015, Vol 60, #7.
[2]Guidelines are appropriate for adult and pediatric populations

PROCEDURES

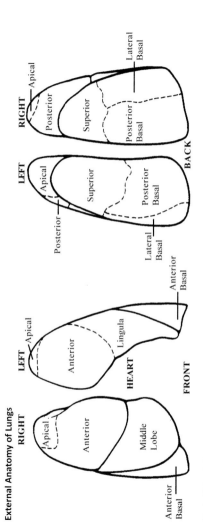

External Anatomy of Lungs

Used with Permission.
An introduction to postural drainage and percussion. In (2012). Cystic Fibrosis Foundation.

Postural Drainage Modified Positions (CFF)

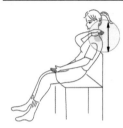

Upper Lobes (Self Percussion)

Patient should sit upright. Instruct pt to percuss area between collarbone and top of shoulderblade, being careful to avoid bony structures.

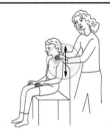

Upper Front Chest

Patient should sit upright. Percuss area between collarbone and top of shoulderblade, being careful to avoid bony structures.

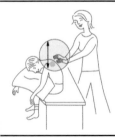

Upper Back Chest

Pt should sit upright, leaning forward at about 30 degrees. Stand behind pt and percuss both sides of upper back, being careful to avoid bony structures.

Used with Permission. Text adapted.

An introduction to postural drainage and percussion. In (2012). Cystic Fibrosis Foundation.

PROCEDURES

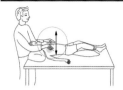

Upper Front Chest

Patient should be supine, with arms to sides. Percuss bilaterally between collarbone and nipple line.

Avoid bony structures and breasts on females.

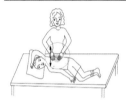

Left Side Front Chest

Patient should be on right side, with left arm over head if able. Percuss over lower ribs, just below nipple line on front of chest.

Avoid abdomen and breasts on females.

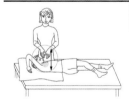

Right Side Front Chest

Patient should be on left side, with right arm over head if able. Percuss over lower ribs, just below nipple line on front of chest.

Avoid abdomen and breasts on females

Used with Permission. Text adapted.

An introduction to postural drainage and percussion. In (2012). Cystic Fibrosis Foundation.

PROCEDURES

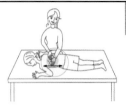

Lower Back Chest

Patient should be proned. Percuss bilaterally at bottom of chestwall (use bottom edge of ribcage as a guide)

Avoid bony stuctures (lower ribcage and vertebral column)

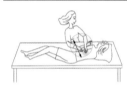

Left Lower Side Back Chest

Pt should be positioned on right side, rolled forward 1/4 turn. Percuss lower left side of chest above bottom edge or ribs

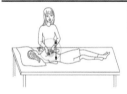

Right Lower Side Back

Patient should be positioned on left side, rolled forward 1/4 turn. Percuss lower right side of chest above bottom edge of ribs

PROCEDURES

Used with Permission. Text adapted.

An introduction to postural drainage and percussion. In (2012). Cystic Fibrosis Foundation.

Traditional Postural Drainage Positions

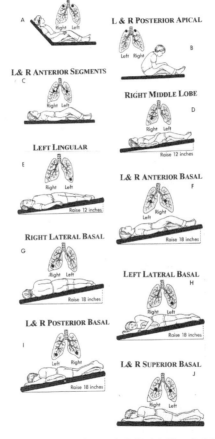

Adapted from Hirsch, J. and Hannock, L. *Mosby's Manual of Clinical Nursing Practice.* Copyright 1985 by Mosby.

Potential Effects of a Head-Down Position

- Aggravation of GERD
- Bronchospasm
- Cardiovascular Changes/Hypotension
- Decreased Maximum Expiratory Pressures and PEF
- Decreased oxygenation
- Discomfort or Pain
- Pts with anxiety sometimes struggle with unusual positioning
- Gastrostomy tube aspiration
- Poor tolerance
- Raised Intracranial Pressure (ICP)
- Rib fractures
- Reduced Vital Capacity (Stomach Pressing on diaphragm, impeding lung expansion)
- Shortness of Breath (SOB)
- Uncomfortable
- V/Q Changes

General Considerations for Airway Clearance Techniques

- Most patients breath and cough better when sitting up, leaning slightly forward (head and neck upright, not bent over).
- A pillow held firmly against the abdomen may permit a stronger cough.
- If inspirations are inadequate, teach diaphragmatic breathing or assist with manual bagging or IPPB/NIV.
- Pain medication should be used as prescribed when pain is a limiting factor.
- Patients should be encouraged to drink more water when secretions are extremely thick (unless on fluid restrictions).

Prior treatment with bronchodilators for bronchospasm, mucolytics/saline/ hypertonic saline may also help aid clearance when secretions are thick and sticky.

- Quadriplegics can use glossopharyngeal breathing or "frog breathing" to improve cough and usually cough better with head of bed flat and often in a side-lying position

In-Exsufflator (Cof-flator™ or Cough Assist™)	
Description	Applies a positive pressure to the airway (mask or tube) and then rapidly shifts to a negative pressure producing a high expiratory flow rate from the lungs stimulating a cough.
Indications	The inability to effectively cough or clear secretions as a result of reduced peak expiratory flow rates (< 5-6 L/s) as seen in high spinal cord injuries, neuro-muscular conditions, or fatigue associated with intrinsic lung disorders.
Contraindications	• Bullous emphysema, recent barotrauma, or patients prone to pneumothorax or pneumomediastinum. • Patients with CV instability should be monitored for SpO_2 and HR.
Directions for use	• Patients usually given 4 - 5 coughing cycles in succession, followed by a 30 second rest period. • There are usually 6 - 10 cycles for a full treatment. • A typical cycle consists of the following: • The unit slowly builds up positive pressure in the chest over a 1 - 3 sec period to about + 40 mm Hg. • It then rapidly switches to the "exhale" mode with a drop in pressure to – 40 mm Hg in 0.02 seconds (total drop of 80 mm Hg). • Exhalation pressure is usually held for 2-3 sec. • This results in a cough and expectoration of secretions. • The device can be titrated to maximum insufflation by chest wall excursion, BS, and patient comfort. • Some models allow for "Manual" versus "Automatic" modes. In automatic mode, Inspiratory and Expiratory Times and Pressures are set as well as a Pause in between breaths. In Manual Mode, Pressures are set, while timing is via switching from Inspiration to Expiration - Breathing at the same rate with the patient can be helpful in synchronizing. May be used by mouthpiece or mask, as well as by tracheostomy.

PROCEDURES

Positive Expiratory Pressure (PEP) Therapy	
Description	Positive expiratory pressure (PEP therapy) is the active exhalation against a variable flow resistor reaching pressures of ~ 10-20 cm H_2O.
Indications	PEP Therapy enhances bronchial hygiene therapy by improving airway patency and airflow through airways that are partially obstructed by stenting the airways and/or increasing intrathoracic pressure distal to retained secretions, which: • Reduces air-trapping in susceptible patients • Promotes increased mobilization and clearance of secretions from the airways • Enhances collateral ventilation and opens airways behind mucus obstructions, improving pulm. mech. & facilitating gas exchange Secondarily, it may help prevent or reverse atelectasis, prevent recurrent infection, and slow disease progression.
Devices	Often a disposable, single-patient use device that is self-administered. It is less time-consuming and does not require the precise positioning of chest physical therapy. Used with FET ("huff coughing").
Procedure	1. Instruct to sit upright, with a tight seal around mouthpiece/mask, then inhale, using the diaphragm, to a volume > VT (but not TLC). 2. Instruct to exhale actively, but not forcefully, to FRC, achieving an airway pressure of 10-20 cm H_2O*. I:E ratio 1:3, 1:4 3. Perform 10-20 breaths through the device, then 2-5 huff coughs. 4. Repeat cycle 5-10 times (15-20 minutes) or until secretions are cleared. *The amount of PEP varies with the size of the adjustable orifice and the level of expiratory flow generated by the patient. Adjust to meet patient's need.
Oscillatory PEP	The combination of PEP therapy with airway vibrations or oscillations. See Hig Frequency Oscillations on following pages.

Use of Positive Airway Pressure Adjuncts to Bronchial Hygiene Therapy[1, 2, 3]

Indications

Aid in mobilizing secretions (CF, CB)

Optimize bronchodilator delivery

Prevent/reverse atelectasis

Reduce air trapping (asthma, COPD)

Contraindications

Relative: active hemoptysis, acute sinusitis, epistaxis, esophageal surgery, hemodynamic instability, ICP (> 20 mm Hg), middle air problems, nausea, recent surgery (facial, oral, or skull), unable to tolerate (↑WOB), untreated pneumothorax.

Frequency

Critical care: q 1-6 hrs

Acute/domiciliary care: 2-4 x/ day or as needed.

Hazards/Complications

Air swallowing (vomit/aspiration), CV compromise (↓ venous return or ischemia), claustrophobia, ↑ ICP, ↑WOB (hypoventilation /hypercarbia), pulmonary barotrauma, skin breakdown/discomfort.

Monitoring

ABG's/O2 Sat, BS, CV parameters (BP, HR, rhythm), ICP, mental function, RR and pattern, skin color, sputum production (qty, color, consistency, odor), subjective response (pain, dyspnea, discomfort, etc.).

Clinical Goals

↑ sputum production, improved ABG's, BS, chest x-ray, ease of secretion clearance, O2 Sat, &/or vital signs.

1) PAP is bronchial hygiene therapy using PEP, EPAP, or CPAP as adjuncts to help mobilize secretions and treat atelectasis.

Positive expiratory pressure (PEP therapy) = exhalation against a fixed orifice resistor reaching pressures of approximately 10-20 cm H_2O.

Expiratory positive airway pressure (EPAP therapy) = exhalation against a threshold resistor reaching preset pressures of 10-20 cm H_2O.

Continuous positive airway pressure (CPAP therapy) = inspiration and expiration within a pressurized circuit and against a threshold resistor maintaining preset pressures of 5-20 cm H_2O.

2) Adapted from the AARC Clinical Practice Guideline: Use of Positive Airway Pressure Adjuncts to Bronchial Hygiene Therapy, *Respiratory Care*, Vol. 38, #5, 1993.

3) Patients should take larger than normal breaths then exhale actively, but not forcefully, creating a positive airway pressure of 10 to 20 cm H_2O. I:E ratio 1:3. Perform 10 - 20 breaths, huff cough 2-3 times, then rest as needed.

Repeat cycle 4-8 times, not to exceed 20 min.

See Following Pages for Detailed Information on Devices

Airway Oscillations

Patient Generated	*Oscillatory PEP Therapy*	The patient's active exhalation through a device performs the work of creating oscillations which are transferred to the patient's airway.
	Acapella, Flutter, Lung Flute, Quake	
Device Generated	*Intrapulmonary Percussive Ventilation (IPV)*	A device which creates short, rapid inspiratory flow pulses into the airway. Expiration is passive from chest wall elastic recoil.
	MetaNeb, Percussionator, PercussiveNeb, IMP2	

Chest Wall Oscillations

Device Generated	*High Frequency Chest Wall Compression (HFCWC)* *Vest/Cuirass*	A device which creates short, rapid expiratory flow pulses in the airway by compressing the chest wall externally. Chest wall elastic recoil returns lung to FRC.
	The Vest, SmartVest, InCourage	
	High Frequency Chest Wall Oscillation (HFCWO)	A device which creates short, rapid biphasic (positive & negative) pressure changes (oscillations) on the chest wall externally, which is transferred to the airway.
	Hayek Oscillator	

PROCEDURES

Description	A disposable, single-patient use device (self-administered) that delivers positive expiratory pressure with high frequency oscillations. Vibratory positive Expiratory Pressure Therapy
Directions	Pt exhales air through an opening that is periodically closed by a pivoting cone. As air passes through the opening, the cone will open and close the airflow path. This produces a vibratory pressure waveform - allowing secretions to be mobilized and expectorated.
Settings	Dial on end of device sets vibration/oscillation frequency (6-20 Hz). Device is available in three flow rate ranges.

Description	A device which produces oscillations in expiratory pressure and airflow. The resultant vibration of the airways loosens mucus from the airway walls.
Contraindications	Patients with Pneumothorax or Right Heart Failure
Directions	• Patient seated with back straight, head tilted slightly back or seated with elbows resting on a table with head tilted slightly back. • Initially, stem is positioned horizontally. Then adjusted up or down to get the maximum "fluttering" effect within the patient's chest (Vibrations can be felt by placing one hand on back and the other on the front of chest). • Patient takes a deep breath (but not to TLC), holds for 2-3 seconds, then exhales actively (but not forcefully) as long as possible while keeping cheeks as hard and flat as possible. • Exhale repeatedly through the device until coughing is stimulated. • Continue for approx. 15 minutes or until patient feels no additional mucus can be raised. • Perform procedure 2-4 times/day or as directed.

Intrapulmonary Percussive Ventilation™ (IPV)

Description	The delivery of high-frequency percussive breaths (sub-tidal volume) into the patient's airways by a pneumatic device.
Indications	The inability to effectively cough or clear secretions as a result of reduced peak expiratory flow rates.
Contra-indications	Bronchospasm, lung contusion, pneumothorax, pulmonary hemorrhage, subcutaneous emphysema, TB, vomiting and aspiration.
Directions	• Pt breathes through a mouthpiece or artificial airway and the unit delivers high flow rate bursts of gas into the lungs from 100-300 x/min. Continuous positive pressure is maintained (typically 15-40 cm H_2O) while the pulses dilate the airways. At the end of the percussive inspiratory cycle (5-10 sec), a deep exhalation is performed with expectoration of secretions. • Normal treatment time is 20 min. Aerosols (Bland or Medicated) may also be delivered via the attached nebulizer with this therapy.
Settings	• Pressure is set via a manometer with optimum range being 30-40 cmH2O (less for ↑ Compliance, more for ↓ Compliance). This is equivalent to setting a "Mean Airway Pressure" • Difficulty knob changes the frequency of the oscillations, which may improve clearance and recruitment. It is recommended that this knob be turned back and forth every few minutes during tx.
Notes	• This therapy can be done as an adjunct to Mechanical Ventilation • Very Important: Circuit configurations are different for ventilator versus non-vented, and should be assembled carefully • When effective, several breaks may need to be taken in order to get pt to cough or suction. • Many clinicians recommend utilizing an inline suction catheter when used in conjunction with an artificial airway to facilitate suctioning. • Cuffed artificial airways: Sx above cuff, and then at least partially deflate cuff during tx to facilitate secretion clearance.

Vest Airway Clearance System™	
Description	• The system includes an air pulse generator, inflatable vest, and connecting tube. • It provides high frequency chest wall compressions which help mobilize secretions.
Indications	• Follow the guidelines established by the AARC for airway clearance therapies. • A patient-specific assessment should always be used weighing potential benefits and risks. • Indications include cystic fibrosis, bronchiectasis, or conditions where the patient has the inability to effectively mobilize and expectorate secretions.
Contra-indications	Active hemorrhage, cardiac instability, chest wall pain, lung contusion, recent thoracic skin grafts, recently placed pacemaker, subQ emphysema, suspected TB, unstabilized head and/or neck injury.
Directions	• As the patient wears the inflatable vest, small gas volumes alternately flow into and out of the unit – rapidly inflating and deflating (compressing and releasing) the chest wall to create air flow and cough- like shear forces to move secretions. • Timing of the pulse is manually controlled by the patient or clinician • The intensity (25-40 mm Hg) and frequency (5-25 Hz) of the pulses can also be adjusted by the patient or clinician • Vests come in various styles (full chest vest down to simple wrap around chest), disposable/nondisposable, and sizes. Ensuring a proper fit and style helps ensure better pt compliance with therapy.

Bronchial Hygiene Selection Algorithm

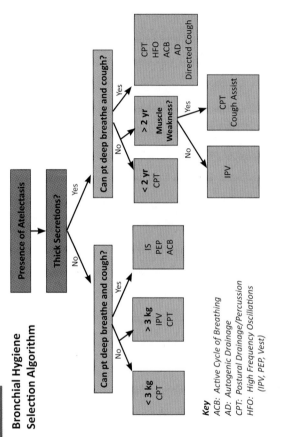

Key

ACB: Active Cycle of Breathing
AD: Autogenic Drainage
CPT: Postural Drainage/Percussion
HFO: High Frequency Oscillations
(IPV, PEP, Vest)

Summary Recommendations by the ACCP*

Autogenic Drainage

Should be taught as an adjunct to postural drainage for patients with CF . . . can be performed without assistance and in one position.

Chest Physical Therapy

Recommended in CF patients as an effective technique to increase mucus clearance. The effects of each treatment are relatively modest and the long-term benefits are unproven.

Cough Assist

Mechanical cough assist devices are recommended in pts with NM disease w/ impaired cough, prevents respiratory complications.

Expiratory Muscle Training

Recommended in patients with NM weakness and impaired cough, to improve peak exp. pressure, which may benefit cough.

High Frequency Techniques

Devices designed to oscillate gas in the airway, either directly or by compressing the chest wall, can be considered as an alternative to chest physiotherapy for patients with CF.

Huff Cough

Huff coughing should be taught as an adjunct to other methods of sputum clearance in patients with COPD and CF.

Manually-Assisted Cough

Should be considered in patients with expiratory muscle weakness to reduce the incidence of respiratory complications. Manually assisted cough may be detrimental and should not be used in persons with airflow obstruction caused by disorders like COPD.

Positive Expiratory Pressure Therapy

Recommended in patients with CF over conventional chest physio-therapy, because it is approximately as effective as chest physiotherapy, and is inexpensive, safe, and can be self-administered.

"The effect of nonpharmacologic airway clearance techniques on long-term outcomes such as health-related quality of life and rates of exacerbations, hospitalizations, and mortality is not known at this time."

* Nonpharmacologic Airway Clearance Therapies: ACCP Evidence-Based Clinical Practice Guidelines, *Chest*. 2006; 129:250S-259S.

PROCEDURES

Notes:

Humidity Therapy

Variable	Considerations
Indications	**Primary Indications** • Humidify dry medical gases (> 4 L/min) • Overcome humidity deficit when upper airway is bypassed **Secondary Indications** • Treat bronchospasm due to cold air • Treat hypothermia • Thickened secretions
Therapeutic Modalities	Used specifically with the following modalities: • Oxygen therapy (esp. when >4 L/min is delivered) • Non-invasive positive pressure ventilation (CPAP and BiPAP ventilation) • Invasive positive pressure ventilation • Artificial Airways via collar or T-Piece
Under-Humidification	• Atelectasis (mucus plugging) • Dry, nonproductive cough • Subsernal pain • Thick, dehydrated secretions • Hypoxemia • ↑ Airway Resistance • ↑ Infection • ↑ WOB
Over-Humidification	• Fluid overload • Pulmonary edema • Surfactant alteration • Thermal damage to mucosa • ↑ Airway secretions (↑airway resistance) • Atelectasis • Hypoxemia
Heat	• Heated Humidification is recommended for artificial airways, thick secretions, and/or patient comfort

Humidification Devices

Type	Use	Comments
Low Flow		
Bubble Diffuser	Used with low flow devices (>4 L/m) and AEM masks (> 50%)	Provides only 20% to 40% of body humidity, may be heated to deliver 100% humidity (and with low flows >7 L/m), should not be used for patients with ET tube or tracheostomy.
High Flow		
Cascade Humidifier	Mainstream "bubble" humidifier for patients with ET tube or tracheostomy.	100% humidity and body temperature. Correct water level is required.
Passover Humidifier	Used for either low or high flow devices (CPAP/ BiPAP) and ventilators.	Effective humidity only when heated to body humidity.
Wick Humidifier	Mainstream "passover" using a porous hygroscopic "wick" to ↑ surface area.	100% humidity and body temperature.
Heat/Moisture Exchanger (HME) (Hygroscopic condenser humidifier [HCH] or artificial nose)	Mainstream "passover" reservoir containing hygroscopic material. Short-term use only with MV (≤ 5 days) *Additional info can be found in Oakes' Mechanical Ventilation Pocket Guide.	Condenses and "traps" exhaled heat and moisture and then evaporates and warms and humidifies (= 70% BH) the inhaled gas. Exchange daily or per manufacturer's recommendations -- Monitor sputum viscosity.
Room Humidifier (cool mist, steam vaporizer, centrifugal)	Used to humidify the room.	Produces 100% humidity at room temperature when in a closed area. Should not be used with ET tube or trach.

Notes (from opposite page):

Distilled or sterile water should be used in bubble humidifiers.
Monitor patient's quantity and quality of airway secretions.

HME: Inspect regularly for partial or complete obstruction by secretions, especially useful during transporting or weaning MV patients.

Heated Humidifier

- Close monitoring of operating and output temperatures, adequate water supply/proper level, and condensation buildup is required.
- Prevent inadvertent tracheal lavage from the condensate.
- Check that alarms are set and working properly

Humidification during Invasive and Noninvasive Mechanical Ventilation[1] (AARC Expert Reference-Based Guideline)

Indication	Hazards/Complications
Mandatory with ET tube or Trach Tube. Optional with NIV (use HH if humidifying)	Burns (patient or caregiver)(HH) Electrical shock (HH) Hypo/hyperthermia Hypoventilation (HME → ↑VD) ↑ Resistive WOB through humidifier Infection (nosocomial) Tracheal lavage (pooled condensate or overfilling) (HH) Underhydration (mucous impaction or plugging of airways → air-trapping, hypoventilation, ↑ WOB) Ventilator malperformance: pooled condensate → ↑ airway pressures or asynchrony with patient (HH) HME → ineffective low pressure alarm during disconnection
Contraindication	
None except **HME** when: Body temperature < 32°C, low VT strategies, expired VT < 70% of delivered VT, spont V̇E > 10 L/min, thick, copious, or bloody secretions.	
Monitoring	
Check: alarm settings (30 – 41°C) (HH), humidifier temp setting (HH), inspired gas temp (34-40°C) (HH), water level and feed system (HH), sputum quantity and consistency Remove condensate in circuit Replace HMEs contaminated with secretions	
	Clinical Goal
	Humidified and warmed inspired gases without hazards or complications.
Frequency:	
Continuous during gas therapy	

1) Adapted from AARC Clinical Practice Guideline: Humidification during Inasive and Noninvasive Mechanical Ventilation, **Respiratory Care**, Vol. 57, #5, 2012.
HH = heated humidity, HME = heat moisture exchanger

PROCEDURES

Lung Expansion Therapy

Variable	Considerations	
Indications	Risk for, or evidence of Atelectasis (usually secondary to pt either not taking deep breaths, or unable to)	
	Passive Atelectasis	Persistent use of small Tidal Volumes (anesthesia, rib fx, drugs, fatigue, immobilitiy, NM disorders, pain, surgery)
	Resorptive Atelectasis	Ventilation blocked by foreign body, mucus plugs, lesion, or spasm
Clinical Signs	• **History:** • Recent abdominal or thoracic surgery • COPD or cigarette smoking • Prolonged bed rest • Morbid Obesity • ↑ **RR, ↑ HR** • **Auscultation:** • Crackles (fine) • Bronchial (consolidation) • ↓ BS (blocked airways) • **CXR:** • ↓ volumes • Opacity • Air bronchograms • Elevated diaphragm • Tracheal shift (severe)	

Minimally Intensive (Self)	• Encourage Deep Breaths
(Device)	• Incentive Spirometry • PEP Therapies (Acapella, Flutter) - see Airway Clearance Section
Intensive (Device + Time)	• Intermittent Pos Pressure Breathing (IPPB) • Intrapercussive Ventilation (IPV) - see Airway Clearance Section • Continuous Positive Airway Pressure (CPAP)
Most Inten	• Therapeutic Bronchoscopy (resorptive)

Incentive Spirometry (IS)	
Description	• Device which encourages deep breathing, usually with measurement (mL) of breath size, as well as indicator of speed (slow is more effective)
Technique	• Designed to mimic natural sigh breaths, by encouraging patients to take slow, deep diaphragmatic inspirations (performing an IC from FRC to near TLC), followed by 5-10 sec breath hold. • Pt should be sitting upright to be most effective. • Directions should be intentionally worded (put the mouthpiece in your mouth, and then take a slow deep breath in like you're drinking a milkshake from a straw). Demonstration may assist in learning. • Set realistic goals, but ones that encourage pt to keep pushing further. • Patient should exhale normally and then rest as long as necessary between maneuvers (prevents resp alkalosis) • Each session should contain a minimum of 5-10 breaths, generally with a minimum of 10 breaths/hour.
Notes	• For post-surgical use, it is best to teach technique prior to surgery and have pt practice (it is more difficult to teach a new skill with pain medication interfering). • Device should be placed in plain sight and reach of pt. Instruct family and/or other available staff to assist in encouraging compliance. • For pts that struggle with technique/coordination, consider instead on focusing on key elements without device - deep, slow breaths with 5-10 second hold.

Incentive Spirometry[1,2]
(AARC Expert Panel Reference-Based Guideline)

Indications

Screen at-risk pts for Post-Op Complications:

Preop screening to obtain baseline*

Atelectasis or predisp. for*:
Surgery (upper/lower abdom, thoracic, COPD, prolonged bedrest, lack of pain control, restrictive lung defect (dysfunctional diaphragm or muscles, NM disease, SCI), sickle cell, CABG

*See also recommendations below

Contraindications

Patient unable or unwilling to use device appropriately (including young pts, delirium, heavy sedation)

Patient unable to take deep breath (VC < 10 mL/kg or IC < 1/3 predicted)

Hazards/Complications

Fatigue

Hyperventilation

Inappropriate (as sole tx for major collapse/consolidat)

Ineffective (if used incorrectly)

Hypoxemia (O2 therapy interrupt)

Pain

Monitoring

Initial instruction and observation of proper performance.

Periodic observation for:
compliance, frequency, number of breaths/session, volume or flow goals (improvement), effort, motivation, device availability,

Suggested Frequencies

10 breaths q. 1-2 hr - awake

10 breaths - 5x/day

15 breaths q. 4 hrs

Outcome Assessment

Decreased atelectasis –
BS improved, fever resolved, ↑oxygenation, reduced FIO2 requirement, improved chest x-ray, pulse rate normal, respiratory rate ↓

See Next Page for Evidence-Based Recommendations
(based on GRADE scoring system)

1) IS is a component of bronchial hygiene therapy designed to encourage spontaneous breathing patients to take long, slow, deep breaths and hold them for ≥3 seconds (sustained maximal inspiration, SMI). The primary purpose is to help maintain airway patency and prevent/reverse atelectasis.

2) Adapted from the AARC Clinical Practice Guideline: Incentive Spirometry, *Respiratory Care*, Volume 56, #10, 2011.

PROCEDURES

AARC Evidence-Based Recommendations: IS
 (based on GRADE system)

- Incentive spirometry alone is **not** recommended for routine use in the preoperative and postoperative setting to prevent postoperative pulmonary complications.
- It **is** recommended that incentive spirometry be used with deep breathing techniques, directed coughing, early mobilization, and optimal analgesia to prevent postoperative pulmonary complications.
- It **is** suggested that deep breathing exercises provide the same benefit as incentive spirometry in the preoperative and postoperative setting to prevent postoperative complications
- Routine use of incentive spirometry to prevent atelectasis in patients after upper-abdominal surgery is **not** recommended
- Routine use of incentive spirometry to prevent atelectasis after coronary artery bypass graft surgery is **not** recommended.
- It **is** suggested that a volume-oriented device be selected as an incentive spirometry device.

Intermittent Positive Pressure Breathing (IPPB)

Goal	• An augmented Vᴛ, achieved with min. effort
Technique	• A semi-Fowler's position is preferred; supine is acceptable when an upright position is contraindicated. • Effectiveness is usually dependent on proper patient instruction and demonstration. • Use mouthpiece/noseclips - mask as last resort. • Optimal breathing pattern is slow, deep breaths held at end-inspiration. • Resulting volumes should be measured and pressure adjusted according to needs and response. • Note: To be effective, Deliv VT > Pt spont efforts • Bland aerosols (NSS) can be delivered via IPPB, but more often, medicated aerosols consisting of a bronchodilator, mucoactive or combination are used. • Treatments usually last 15 - 20 minutes.

Common Goals and Settings	Parameter	Suggested Goal/Setting
	Sensitivity	1-2 cmH₂O (easy trigger, but no autocycle)
	Pressure	Initial: 10-15 cmH2O Goal: set to Target Vᴛ (see below)
	Target Vol.	10-15 cc/kg PBW (30% pred. IC)
	Rate	6 breaths/min
	I:E Ratio	1:3 to 1:4

Trouble-shooting	Large negative Pressure swings	Incorrect sensitivity: set to autotrigger, then decrease sens until pt able to trigger easily
	↓ Press after insp. begins, or failure to rise until breath's end	Inspiratory flow too low
	Premature cycle off	Insp flow too high or airflow obstructed (kinked tubing, occluded mouthpiece, active resistance to inhalation)
	Failure to cycle off	Leak (neb, exhalation, pt interface, nose)

IPPB[1,2]
(AARC Expert Panel Reference-Based Guideline)

Indications

Lung expansion –
Atelectasis (when not responsive to other therapies or patient can't/won't cooperate)
Secretions (inability to clear)

Short-term ventilation (alternative form of MV for hypoventilating patients, consider NPPV)

Delivery of aerosolized medication[3] –
Used when other aerosol techniques have been unsuccessful.[4]
Patients with fatigue, severe hyperinflation or during short-term ventilation.

Assessment of Need

Acute, severe, unresponsive bronchospasm/ COPD exac.
Impending respiratory failure
NM disorders
PFT (FEV1 < 65% pred, FVC < 70% pred, MVV < 50% pred, VC < 10 mL/kg) w/o eff cough
Significant atelectasis

Contraindications

Absolute – untreated tension pneumothorax
Relative – active hemoptysis, active untreated TB, air swallowing, bleb, hemo instability, hiccups, ICP > 15 mm Hg, nausea, recent oral, facial, esophageal or skull surgery, TE fistula.

Monitoring

Patient: RR, V_T, HR, rhythm, BP, BS, response (mental function, pain, discomfort, dyspnea), skin color, O_2 Sat, sputum, ICP, chest x-ray.
Machine: f, V_T, peak, plateau, PEEP pressures, sensitivity, flow, FIO_2, T_I, T_E.

Clinical Goals

For lung expansion: a V_T of at least 33% of IC predicted
↑ FEV_1 or PF
More effective cough, enhanced secretion clearance, improved chest x-ray and BS, good patient response.

Hazards/Complications

Air trapping (auto PEEP), barotrauma, ↓venous return, exacerbation of hypoxemia, gastric distention, hemoptysis, hyperoxia (with O_2), hypocarbia, hypo / hyperventilation, ↑Raw, V/Q mismatch, infection, psychological dependence, secretion impaction.

Frequency

Critical care: q 1-6 hrs as tolerated, re-evaluate daily

Acute care: bid to 4 times per day per patient response, re-evaluate q 24 hrs

SEE NOTES NEXT PAGE

NOTES (from Previous Page)

1) Intermittent positive pressure breathing (IPPB) is intermittent, or short-term mechanical ventilation for the purpose of augmenting lung expansion, assisting ventilation, and/or delivering an aerosolized medication (not the therapy of first choice) (Does not include NPPV).

2) Adapted from the AARC Clinical Practice Guideline: IPPB, 2003 Revision + Update, *Respiratory Care*, Volume 48, #5, 2003.

3) Efficacy is technique dependent (coordination, breathing pattern, VI, PIP, inspiratory hold), device design, and patient instruction.

4) MDI or nebs are devices of choice for aerosol therapy to COPD or stable asthma patients.

Oxygen Therapy

Therapeutic Gases

Cylinder Color Standards, by Gas

Gas	USA	ISO*
Oxygen (O_2)	GREEN	WHITE
Air	YELLOW/SILVER	WHITE/BLACK
Carbon dioxide (CO_2)	GRAY	GRAY
CO_2 and O_2	GRAY/GREEN	GRAY/WHITE
Helium (He)	BROWN	BROWN
He and O_2	BROWN/GREEN	BROWN/WHITE
Nitrous Oxide (N_2O)	BLUE	BLUE
Cyclopropane (C_3H_6)	ORANGE	ORANGE
Ethylene (C_2H_4)	RED	VIOLET
Nitrogen	BLACK	BLACK

*ISO: International Standards Organization

SEE ALSO:

Oxygen Blending Ratios	See pg 9-28
Oxygen Entrainment Ratios	see pg 9-30
Oxygen Duration Times	see pg 9-29
Oxygen Assessment Equations	see pg 9-4

PROCEDURES

E-Cylinder (O₂) Estimated Tank Duration in Minutes *(no reserve)**
(0.28 x PSI / LPM)

LPM	Pressure (PSI)							
	500 (reserve)	750	1,000	1,250	1,500	1,750	2,000	2,200
1	140	210	280	350	420	490	560	616
2	70	105	140	175	210	245	280	308
3	46	70	93	116	140	163	186	205
4	35	52	70	87	105	122	140	154
5	28	42	56	70	84	98	112	123
6	23	35	46	58	70	81	93	102
10	14	21	28	35	42	49	56	61
12	11	17	23	29	35	40	46	51
15	09	14	18	23	28	32	37	41

H-Cylinder (O₂) Estimated Tank Duration in Minutes *(no reserve)**
(3.14 x PSI/LPM)

LPM	Pressure (PSI)							
	500 (reserve)	750	1,000	1,250	1,500	1,750	2,000	2,200
1	1570	2355	3140	3925	4710	5495	6280	6908
2	785	1177	1570	1962	2355	2747	3140	3454
3	523	785	1046	1308	1570	1831	2093	2302
4	392	588	785	981	1177	1373	1570	1727
5	314	471	628	785	942	1099	1256	1381
6	261	392	523	654	785	915	1046	1151
10	157	235	314	392	471	549	628	690
12	130	196	261	327	392	457	523	575
15	104	157	209	261	314	366	418	460

*These charts represent total duration with no Reserve. Best Clinical practice dictates not including the last 500 PSI in your calculation (this is emergency reserve).

See Chapter 9 for Detailed Oxygen Duration Equations

Oxygen Monitoring

Method	Normal Values	Description
Noninvasive		
SpO_2	> 95%	Peripheral O_2 saturation (measured Hb saturation via Pulse Oximeter)
TCM	~80-100 mm Hg	Transcutaneous Monitoring estimates PaO_2 by inducing hyperperfusion (via heating) of skin site, and measures electrochemically
Invasive		
PaO_2	80 -100 mm Hg	Partial Pressure of Oxygen molecules within blood (not those bound to hemoglobin)
SaO_2	95-95%	Calculated O_2 saturation from PaO_2 (if an analysis), or actual measured value (co-oximeter)

Notes:
- Trends are more important than absolute values.
- SpO_2 may be a poor indicator of SaO_2
- Periodic baseline correlations should be made with PaO_2 and/or SaO_2 (CO-oximetry).
- Pulse oximetry alone can not indicate hyperoxemia (maximum is 100%).
- SpO_2 values may vary between various models of oximeters, so caution in interchanging oximeters on same pt
- Factors affecting SpO_2 – See also Next Page

Noninvasive Monitoring

See following pages

Pulse Oximetry[1, 2]

Indications
Need to monitor SaO_2, need to quantitate patient's response to therapy or diagnostic procedure.

Contraindications
Ongoing need to measure pH, $PaCO_2$, total Hgb, and or abnormal Hgb (relative).

Hazards/Complications
Inappropriate therapy due to false negative or positive results, probe misuse (pressure sores, burns, electrical shock).

Frequency
Variable depending on clinical status, indications, and procedures being performed.

Monitoring
Validity of reading –
Compare SpO_2 with SaO_2 and HR with pulse rate (initial and periodic).
Document conditions: patient position, activity level, assess site perfusion, probe location, type of oxygen therapy.
Check for invalidating factors: abnormal Hgb, exposure to light, hyperoxemia, intra vascular dyes, low perfusion state, motion artifact, nail polish/covering, saturation < 83%, skin pigmentation.

Patient – vital signs

Clinical Goal
(desired outcome)
To reflect the patient's clinical, oxygenation, condition.

[1] Pulse oximetry (SpO_2) is a noninvasive determination of oxyhemoglobin saturation (SaO_2).
[2] Adapted from the AARC Clinical Practice Guideline: Pulse Oximetry, *Respiratory Care*, Vol. 36, #12, 1991

Pulse oximetry is helpful in identifying changes in lung function and establishing the need for a change in or discontinuation of O_2 therapy.

The Respiratory Care Practitioner must be acutely aware of the potential inaccuracies of oximetry readings and take them into account when recommending changes. Never use oximetry results as the only parameter when making respiratory care decisions.

PROCEDURES

Troubleshooting the Pulse Oximeter

Problem	Possible Cause(s)	Interventions
Inaccurate SpO$_2$ (does not correlate with SaO$_2$ from ABG)	**Patient**	
	• Movement*	• Encourage pt to be still, if possible or able
*New pulse oximeters are less likely to cause these problems	• Poor perfusion (cool skin, PVD, etc.)	• Check sensor site - consider moving from one finger to another, earlobe, toe, forehead, nare
	• Skin pigment (darker)*	• Consider replacing sensor
	• High carboxyhemoglobin or methemoglobin	• Use other forms of measure if needed to confirm (ABG, TCM, etc.)
	• Reduced arterial blood flow	• Warm site with approved warming device
	Environment	
	• Cool Room*	• Warm site with approved warming device
	• Ambient Light*	• Cover sensor to block ambient light
	• BP Cuff Placement	• Ensure sensor is not distal to BP cuff
	Equipment	
	• Blood Pressure	• Ensure sensor is placed securely; replace if necessary.
	• Sensor not adhering well	• Check sensor site - consider moving from one finger to another, earlobe, toe, forehead, nare
		• Consider different type of sensor (neonatal, etc.)
		• Use ECG signal synchronization.
		• Select a longer (10-15 sec) averaging time, if possible.

PROCEDURES

Problem	Possible Cause(s)	Interventions
Loss of Pulse Signal, Poor Waveform *New pulse oximeters are less likely to cause these problems	**Patient** • Reduced arterial blood flow • Anemia • Hypothermia • Shock (hypotension, vasocon) • Nail polish*	• Confirm or follow with ABG • Check Hemoglobin level • Consider warming site, replace sensor • Always check pt's condition, Vitals • More likely to intefere if contains metallic flakes, remove
	Environment • Excessive ambient light*	• Cover sensor to block ambient light
	Equipment • Constriction by sensor • Sensor is not on patient	• Check sensor • Move to a different site or change type of sensor used • Confirm sensor is on patient
Inaccurate Pulse Rate	**Patient** • Excessive patient motion	• Encourage pt to be still if possible, or able
	Equipment • Pronounced dicrotic notch on art. waveform • Poor quality ECG signal • Electrocautery interference	• Move sensor to a different site • Check ECG leads; replace if necessary. • Same as above.

Arterial Puncture – See AARC CPG: Sampling for Arterial Blood Gas Analysis, Chapter 2

Arterial Line – See Oakes' Hemodynamic Monitoring: A Bedside Reference Manual for an excellent review of indications, insertion sites, equipment, insertion techniques, maintenance, infection control, drawing a blood sample, pressure and waveform variations, complications, trouble-shooting, and removal of the A-Line.

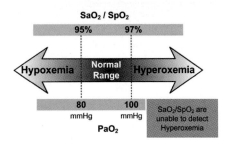

Normal Variations:

Due to FIO_2, barometric pressure, or age

$\quad\quad$ ($PaO_2 \approx 110 - \frac{1}{2}$ patient's age)

SaO_2 = Calculated O_2 saturation from PaO_2 (if an analysis)

$\quad\quad$ (actual measured value if with a co-oximeter)

SpO_2 = Peripheral O_2 saturation (measured value of Hb saturation

$\quad\quad$ with a pulse oximeter).

PaO_2-SaO_2 Relationship

PaO_2	SaO_2*
150	100 %
100	97 %
80	95 %
60	90 %
55	88 %
40	75 %

*varies with shifts in
oxyhemoglobin curve

Always Check for
Proper Correlation between the
PaO_2/SaO_2 calculated values and
the measured SpO_2 value.

PROCEDURES

Oxyhemoglobin Dissociation Curve

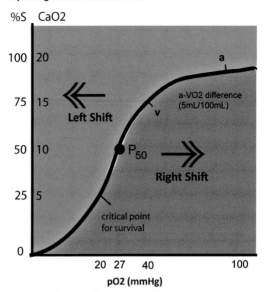

Curve shift = the Bohr effect

a = normal arterial blood

v = normal venous blood

P_{50} = PaO_2 @ 50% Saturation (normal = 27 mmHg)

Left Shift (↑ Hgb-O_2 affinity; ↓ P_{50})	Right Shift (↓ Hgb-O_2 affinity; ↑ P_{50})

Alkalosis
Decreased: temp, PCO_2,
  PO^4, 2,3 DPG (stored
  blood)
Polycythemia
Abnormal Hgb (Fetal Hgb,
HgbCo, metHgb)
	Acidosis
	Increased: temp, PCO_2, PO^4,
	  2,3 DPG
	Anemias (sickle cell)
	Chronic hypoxemia (high altitude)

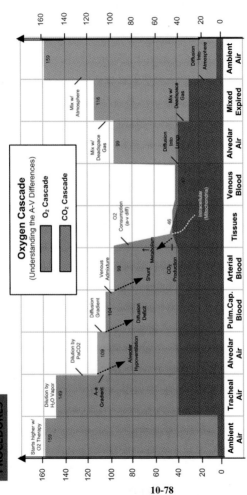

Oxygen Cascade
(Understanding the A-V Differences)

- O₂ Cascade
- CO₂ Cascade

10-78

Assessment of Oxygenation

Oxygenation at the Lungs (external respiration)			Oxygenation at the Tissues (internal respiration)		
	Norm	Ab-norm		Norm	Ab-norm
Adequacy					
PaO_2*	80-100 mmHg	< 80 mmHg	$P\bar{V}O_2$	35-42 mmHg	< 35 or > 45 mmHg
CaO_2	15-24 mL/dL	↑↓	$C\bar{V}O_2$	12-15 mL/dL	↑↓
SaO_2**	> 95%	< 95%	$S\bar{V}O_2$	60-80%	< 60%
SpO_2	> 95%	< 95%	$Ca\text{-}\bar{V}O_2$	4.5-5.0 mL/dL	↑↓
Efficiency					
$PA\text{-}aO_2$	10-25 mmHg (air) 30-50 mmHg (100%)	>25 mmHg	O_{2ER}	25%	↑↓
			$\dot{V}O_2$	200-250 mL/min	↑↓
			$\dot{D}O_2$	750 - 1000 mL/min	↑↓
PaO_2/PAO_2	0.8-0.9	<0.6	VQI	0.8	↑↓
PaO_2/FIO_2	>300	<300			
$PA\text{-}aO_2/PaO_2$	<1.0	>1.0			
Qs/Q_T phys	2-5%	> 20%			

*Normal Variations: Due to age, FIO2, or barometric pressure
Age: PaO2 ≈110 - 1/2 patient's age
**SaO2 = calculated O2 saturation from PaO2
SpO2 = Peripheral O2 saturation - measured value of Hgb saturation with a pulse oximeter.

10-79

Types of Hypoxemia, by Abnormal Values

Types		PAO_2	PaO_2	$PA\text{-}aO_2$	$Pa\text{-}vO_2$	$PaCO_2$	$PACO_2$	$Pa\text{-}ACO_2$
Atmospheric		↓	↓	N	N	↓	↓	N
Tidal		↓	↓	N ↑	N	↑	↑	N
ALVEOLAR	Deadspace	N ↓	N ↓	N↕	N↕	N↕	↓	↑
	Absolute Shunt	N ↑	↓	↑	N	N↕	N↕	N↕
	V/Q Mismatch (relative shunt)	N	↓	↑	N	N↕	N↕	N↕
	Diffusion defect	N	N ↓	↑	N	N ↓	N ↓	N
Hemoglobic		N	N	N	N	N ↓	N ↓	N
Stagnant		N	↓	↑	↑↑	N↕	N↕	N↕
Histotoxic		N	N	N	↓	N	N	N
Demand		*Any of the above*						

For details on values, see Equation Chapter

Hypoxemia

Levels of Hypoxemia

	PaO₂	SpO₂ %	(PaO₂) Clinical Notes
Mild Hypoxemia	60-79 mmHg	90-94%	
Moderate Hypoxemia	40-59 mmHg	75-89%	
Severe Hypoxemia	< 40 mmHg	< 75%	PaO_2 30: loss of consciousness PaO_2 20: anoxia- brain injury likely

Refractory Hypoxemia: Hypoxemia that shows no or little ↑ PaO₂ with ↑ FIO₂. -- Defined as < 5 mmHg ↑ PaO₂ with 0.1 ↑ FIO₂.

Responsive Hypoxemia: Hypoxemia that shows a significant ↑ PaO₂ with ↑ FIO₂. Defined as > 5 mmHg ↑ PaO₂ with 0.1 ↑ FIO₂.

Hypoxemic Respiratory Failure

Known as: Type I Acute Respiratory Failure (ARF), Lung Failure, Oxygenation Failure, or Respiratory Insufficiency

Definition: The failure of the lungs and heart to provide adequate O₂ to meet metabolic needs.

Criteria: PaO₂ < 60 mmHg on FIO₂ ≥ 0.50 -or-
 PaO₂ < 40 mmHg on any FIO₂ -and/or-
 SaO₂ < 90 %

Signs & Symptoms of Acute Hypoxemia/Hypoxia (Relative order of appearance)		Signs & Symptoms of Chronic Hypoxemia/Hypoxia
Tachypnea Dyspnea Pallor Tachycardia Hypertension Headache Anxiety Cyanosis Arrhythmias Blurred or tunnel vision Impaired judgment	Confusion Euphoria Bradycardia Hypotension Nausea/vomiting Loss of coordination Lethargy/weakness Tremors Hyper-active reflexes Stupor Coma ≈ 30 mm Hg Death	Arrhythmias ↓ CO Clubbing (sometimes) Dyspnea Irritability Tiredness Papilledema Polycythemia Impaired judgment Myoclonic jerking Pulmonary hypertension

Types & Causes of Hypoxemia/Hypoxia

Types		Examples
Atmospheric	Insufficient O_2 available	$\downarrow FIO_2$: Drowning (no FIO_2); O_2 therapy error ($\downarrow FIO_2 < 0.21$) $\downarrow PAO_2$: High altitude ($PaO_2 \downarrow 4$ mmHg/1000 ft)
Tidal	Hypoventilation ($\uparrow PaCO_2 \rightarrow \downarrow PaO_2$)	Many causes of pulmonary compromise
Alveolar	1. Deadspace (alveolar) (wasted ventilation; ventilation without perfusion) (V/Q)	$\uparrow$ Alveolar deadspace : a) Complete block: Pulmonary embolus (air, blood, fat, tumor) b) $\downarrow$ blood flow: Shock, cardiac arrest, $\uparrow$ PVR c) $\uparrow V/\downarrow Q$: $\uparrow$ MV and/or PEEP ($\uparrow$ lung zones 1+2 from $\uparrow$ Palv)
	2. Shunt A) Absolute (True) Shunt (Perfusion without ventilation; 0/Q) B) Relative shunt (perfusion with $\downarrow$ ventilation; $\downarrow V/Q$) (V/Q mismatch, shunt effect, or venous admixture)	Anatomical shunts: Pleural, bronchial, thebesian veins, anatomical defects **Capillary shunts +/or Shunt effect:** a) Alveoli collapsed, fluid filled or blocked (complete or partial): ARDS, atelectasis (most common), cystic fibrosis, pneumonia, pneumothorax, pulmonary edema b) $\downarrow$ or no alveolar ventilation: Airway obstruction, asthma, COPD, position changes, secretions, etc.
	3. Diffusion Defect ($\uparrow$ a-c membrane thickness)	Fibrosis, Proteinosis, Sarcoidosis

Types	Causes	Examples
Hemoglobic	Blood abnormality ($\downarrow$ CaO2)	Anemia, hemorrhage, sickle cell, CO poison
		Shift of oxyhemoglobin dissociation curve to right
Stagnant	Blood perfusion abnormality ($\downarrow$ O2 transport)	CV failure, arrythmias, hemorrhage, shock
Histotoxic	Tissue can't metabolize O2	Cyanide poisoning
Demand	$\uparrow$ Metabolic demand for more O2 (which then causes one or more of the above hypoxemic conditions)	Burns, exercise, fever, hyperthyroidism

See Oakes' ABG Pocket Guide: Interpretation and Management for:
• Disinguishing between types of Hypoxemia
• Hypoxemia Diagnostic Algorithm
• Estimating Degree of Pulmonary Dysfunction

ABG Pocket Guide
Interpretation and Management
Dana Oakes

Hypoxemia Diagnostic Algorithm

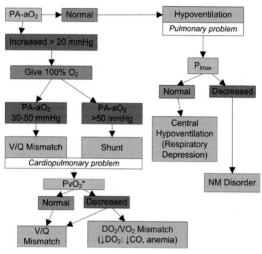

CO = Cardiac Output

* PvO_2 is obtained from a CVP line or PA catheter

OXYGEN THERAPY

Targets for Improving (Correcting) Oxygenation *

	PaO₂ (Goal)	SaO₂/SpO₂ (Goal)
Normal lung	≥80 mmHg	≥95%
Mild lung injury	≥70 mmHg	≥93%
Moderate lung injury	≥60 mmHg	≥90%
Severe lung injury **	≥55 mmHg	≥88%

* Permissive hypoxemia is gaining interest/acceptance when there is concern for O₂ toxicity and/or VILI.

** In shunts with > 50% FIO₂, ↑ FIO₂ has little to no effect. Therefore, in these situations (eg., ARDS) FIO₂ can be lowered to < 50% O₂ to reduce O₂ toxicity to the lungs without compromising PaO₂.

> **See Oakes' ABG Pocket Guide: Interpretation and Management of Oxygenation for:**
> • Evaluating Oxygenation Status
> • Lung Adequacy and Efficiency
> • Estimating Degree of Pulm. Dysfunction
> • Distinguishing Shunts, Deadspace, and Diffusion Defects
> • Assessment of Tissue Oxygen.
> • Management of Oxygenation
> • O2 Therapy for Vented Patients
> • (And More!)

See Equation Chapter for a Complete List of Oxygenation Equations

PROCEDURES

Oxygen Therapy for Adults in the Acute Care Facility[1]
(AARC Expert Panel Evidence-Based Guideline)

Indications

Acute MI

Hypoxemia (actual or suspected)

$PaO_2 < 60$ mm Hg

$SaO_2 < 90\%$

(or below desired) in adults, children, infants > 28 days in room air.

Severe trauma

Short-term therapy or postop

Precautions/Complications

Ventilatory depression: patients on an O_2 drive with elevated $PaCO_2$ and $PaO_2 \geq 60$ mm Hg.

$FIO_2 > 0.5$: absorption atelectasis, ↓ciliary function, ↓leukocyte function, fire hazard, bacterial contamination (humidification system), caution in patients with paraquat poisoning or receiving bleomycin, O_2 toxicity.

Contraindications

Monitoring

Patient:

Clinical assessment (pulm, CV, neuro status)

PaO_2 and/or SaO_2:

Upon initiation of therapy or within –

2 hours (COPD)

8 hours ($FIO_2 > 0.4$)

12 hours ($FIO_2 < 0.4$)

72 hours (acute MI)

Equipment:

q day or more frequent when: $FIO_2 > 0.5$, clinically unstable, heated gas mixture, artificial airway, blending systems.

Frequency

Continuous or intermittent (exercise, sleep)

1) Adapted from the AARC Clinical Practice Guidelines: Oxygen Therapy for Adults in the Acute Care Facility, 2002 Revision & Update *Respiratory Care*, Volume 47, #6, 2002.

OXYGEN DELIVERY DEVICES

Low Flow System (Delivers 100% O_2 at flows < patient's inspiratory (demand). Room air is entrained, total patient demand is not met, and FIO_2 is highly variable.)

Delivery System	Flow, FIO_2	O_2% delivered[1]	Comments	
Nasal Cannula	1-6 L/min	24-40%	Delivers approximately 4%/L, comfortable, good for low %, inexpensive, patient can eat, talk, and sleep.	$\downarrow FIO_2$ as $\dot{V}e\uparrow$, need patient nasal passages, use humidifier ≥ 4 L/min, easily dislodged, may cause irritation, dryness, or nosebleed.
Nasal Catheter	1-6 L/min	24-45%	Same as cannula	Same as cannula, plus must be changed every 8 hours, clogs easily, abdominal distention.
Simple Mask	5-10 L/min	35-50%	Delivers approx. 4%/L, FIO_2 variable depending on fit and ventilation variables., hot/uncomfortable, interferes with eating/talking.	Need minimum 5 L/min to flush CO_2 from mask, more skin irritation
Partial Rebreathing Mask	6-10 L/min	40-70%	High % delivered, same as simple mask, FIO_2 variable depending on fit	$\dot{V}$ should be set to keep reservoir > 1/3 - 1/2 full upon inspiration
Non-Rebreathing Mask	≥ 10 L/min	60-80%	Same as partial rebreathing mask	Same as partial rebreathing mask.

Delivery System		O₂ % delivered¹	Comments
High Flow System (High air flow with oxygen enrichment [HAFOE] which may meet the total demand of the patient [should be ≥ 60 L/min])			
Air Entrainment Mask (Venturi)	Variable	24-50%	Exact O₂ concentrations, can be adapted to deliver aerosol, device of choice for patients on O₂ drive. Entrainment ports easily occluded.

AIR ENTRAINMENT RATIOS

O₂%	Air/O₂ ratio
24%	25/1
28%	10/1
30%	8/1
35%	5/1
40%	3/1

O₂%	Air/O₂ ratio
50%	1.7/1
60%	1/1
70%	0.6/1
80%	0.3/1

Calculating Oxygen Blending Ratios & Entrainment Ratios – See Equations, Chapter 9

| Air Entrainment Nebulizer or High-Volume Humidifier | 8-40 L/min | 28-100% | Used to deliver precise O₂ and/ or aerosol, high O₂%, can provide controlled temperature of gas. FIO2 determined by the nebulization system and flow rate or blender. Use with aerosol mask, face tent, T-piece, trach mask or collar. May need two or three setups to meet inspiratory flow when FIO2 > 50%. Hazards of aerosol therapy. (See aerosol therapy), condensation in tubing. |

Delivery System	Liter flow	O_2% delivered[1]	Comments
High-flow Therapy Systems	Neonatal: 1- 8 L/min	21% - 100%	Used to deliver precise O_2 and humidification from 80% to 100% RH at body temp (37° C). FIO_2 is determined by analysis via bleed-in or blender.
	Pediatric: 8-20 L/min		Beneficial in adults with COPD, pulmonary fibrosis, CHF, asthma, CF and post-surgical care where low-flow oxygen or other delivery systems is inadequate
	Adult: 20-60 L/min	30-100% (variable, dependent on pt flow requirement versus flow delivered)	Can also be used in humidifying CPAP, improving pulmonary hygiene, tracheostomy management and in the treatment of rhinitis/sinusitis.
			Use with a special large-bore nasal cannula to accommodate high liter flows.
			Recommended for neo/ped pts with oxygenation difficulties related to BPD, CF and other pulm conditions w/ PaO_2 <55 mmHg or SpO_2 <88%, tachypnea, retractions, mild apneas and/or bradycardia (AOP).
			Use in conjunction with SpO_2 monitoring
			May create variable CPAP effect (some estimate as much as 1 cmH2O per 10 L/min, though may vary widely by device, physiology, etc.)

1) Based upon AARC Clinical Practice Guideline, Oxygen Therapy for Adults in the Acute Care Facility — 2002 Revision & Update, *Respiratory Care*, Vol 47, # 6, 2002.

PROCEDURES

Oxygen Conserving Devices (OCD)

OCDs provide oxygen on inspiration only, thereby reducing the amount of oxygen used. Due to individual patient variations, prescribed flows must be individually determined by SaO2 during rest and exercise.

Types of OCDs

Type		Disadvantages
Reservoir Cannula "Mustache" or pendant	Least expensive to operate Reduces the amount of oxygen use	Conspicuous Expensive to buy and frequent replacement Heavy/cumbersome Uncomfortable
Pulse-dose or Demand-flow Systems (May be rate responsive)	Reduces the amount of oxygen use Some units switch to continuous flow if inspiration is not detected See * below	Annoying clicking noise If battery-powered, device must be maintained and recharged Cannot be used with oxygen concentrator Catheters and sensors may malfunction Cumbersome Nasal breathing required to trigger (perform nocturnal SpO2)

Continued on Next Page

PROCEDURES

Type	Advantages	Disadvantages
Transtracheal Oxygen System (TTOS) **	Improved compliance Increased mobility Less accidental disruption during sleep; improved sleep Less facial/nasal/ear irritation (vs cannula) May combine with a pulse-dosed oxygen device (oxygen use reduced even more) More cosmetically appealing Reduces the amount of oxygen use Senses of taste and smell are not affected	Catheter dislodgment or lost tract High cost Humidification required Invasive procedure with complications: infection, bleeding, bronchospasm, and subQ emphysema Mucus plugging – requires daily cleaning, saline instillation, and maintenance and periodic replacement Not for all patients Requires significant self-care and patient education

It is not possible to calculate cylinder duration times when OCDs are in use because of 3 variables: cylinder size, setting on OCD regulator, and patient's actual respiratory rate. Most OCDs provide a savings ratio (i.e., 3:1, 4:1), which estimates the improved cylinder duration when compared to the continuous flow setting and helps better predict cylinder duration.

* Pulse-dose systems provide a bolus of O2 at a relatively high flow rate during only the first part of inspiration; demand-flow systems provide oxygen at the set flow throughout the inspiratory phase. Hybrid systems incorporate the features of pulse-dose and demand-flow (a large bolus of oxygen during the initial inspiratory phase followed by oxygen flow throughout the rest of inspiration).

** Indications for TTOS – Problems with standard devices: complications, cosmetics, inadequate oxygenation, need for improved mobility, poor compliance.

Relative contraindications of TTOS – Cardiac arrhythmias, compromised immune system, copious sputum, excessive anxiety, prolonged bleeding times, severe bronchospasm, uncompensated respiratory acidosis.

Heliox Therapy (Helium - Oxygen)

Function	Helium reduces the resistance of air/O_2 flowing through narrowed airways. Its primary value is in the tx of airway obstruction by enhancing the delivery of O_2 and aerosol to the distal areas of the lung. Helium can be used as a temporizing agent to reduce WOB and allow time for the more standard forms of therapy to reach peak effect.
Indications	• Acute exacerbations of COPD or asthma • Post extubation stridor • Status asthmaticus • Tracheal stenosis • Upper airway obstruction

Benefits	• Improved homogeneity of gas distribution resulting in:
	   • ↑ alveolar ventilation, oxygenation and V_T,
	   • ↓ WOB, $PaCO_2$, gas trapping, auto-PEEP, PIP and Pplat, barotrauma, I:E ratios, and shunting
	• Movement of the equal-pressure point of the airways upstream

Common Mixtures	• 80% He / 20% O_2 • 70% He / 30% O_2 * (* Used when O_2 therapy is indicated for hypoxemia. If FIO_2 > 0.6 is required, He/O_2 will have little effect)
Admin-istration	**Spontaneous breathing**: Deliver via tight-fit NRB. May add O_2 nasal cannula to titrate to desired SpO_2. **Intubated**: Deliver as adjunct via ventilator **Delivery using an O_2 flowmeter requires flow conversion:** 70/30: set flow x 1.6 = total flow delivered 80/20: set flow x 1.8 = total flow delivered

Monitoring	ABG sampling Arrhythmia Dyspnea (WOB & SOB)	Heart rate Pulse oximetry Pulsus paradoxus
Hazards	Anoxia- analyze delivered gas Barotrauma- via ventilators not designed for heliox	Too ↑ or too ↓ bronchodilator - too ↓or ↑of a flow through the neb Hypothermia - via hood on infants

11 Diseases and Disorders

CONTENTS

Continued Next Page

These are diseases/disorders commonly found in adults.

- See **Oakes' Neonatal/Pediatric Respiratory Care** for neonatal and pediatric diseases/disorders.
- See **Oakes' Ventilator Management** for ventilation strategies for many of these diseases/disorders.
- See **RespiratoryUpdate.com** for Evidence-Based Guidelines and Expanded Disease Information.

Explanation of Key Used throughout this Chapter

NAME - MOST COMMONLY ACCEPTED MEDICAL TERM LISTED IN ALPHABETICAL ORDER (OTHER NAMES OR ABBREVIATIONS)	
Def	Definition
Types	When present, contains information regarding various types of disease or disorder
	Origin of disease or disease-causing organisms.
CM	**Clinical Manifestations** Listings indicate the most commonly found pulmonary manifestations (not all-inclusive). Manifestations of other body systems are generally not included.
CXR	**Chest X-Ray** - common findings
EBG	**Evidence-Based Guidelines** Available for Topic
CC	**Critical Care Considerations** - note that this will indicate material available in other Oakes' Pocket Guides, as well as online at RespiratoryUpdate.com.
Tx	**Treatment Overview**, including relevant algorithms based on latest Evidence-Based Medicine

Not every category will be presented for every disease - only those that have been deemed clinically relevant.

	ACQUIRED IMMUNE DEFICIENCY SYNDROME (AIDS)
Definition	Infection with human immunodeficiency virus (HIV) which attacks CD4 T-lymphocytes of the immune system to produce a profound **immunosuppressed** state resulting in **opportunistic infections** and Kaposi's sarcoma.
	HIV, plus secondary infections of Pneumocystis, viral, bacterial, or mycoplasma pneumonia, and any other opportunistic infection. High Risk populations include multiple sexual partners, IV drug users, Hemophilia. **Stages**: 1. Viral Transmission 2. Acute HIV Infection 3. Seroconversion (4-10 weeks after viral transmission) 4. Clinical Latent Period (asymptomatic besides possible lymphadenopathy) 5. Early Symptomatic HIV Infection (P. Carinii in up to 50% of cases, bacterial PNA also possible) 6. AIDS (CD4 < 200 mm3 - symptomatic or asymptomatic) 7. Advanced HIV Infection (CD4 < 50 mm3) - 12-18 mos survival usually at this time
CM	Variable depending on cause of infection. Usually ↓ WBC, lymphocytes, and CD4 T cells (the lower the cell count, the greater the severity of infection).
CXR	Variable depending on type of infection. Note that CXR may be normal in pts with HIV who have no active secondary infection.
Tx	**Primary**: Antiretroviral Therapies Goals center around treating HIV viruses (HARRT) and aggressively addressing secondary infections. Current trends favor identifying specific causes of infection and treating those (versus empiric therapies).

ACTINOMYCOSIS

Def

Chronic suppurative and granulomatous fungal infection which may cause pneumonia. It presents in three anatomic forms (1) cervicofacial, (2) thoracic, and (3) abdominal.

Actinomyces israelii (not a true fungus) Gram+ rod, anaerobic.

Route: aspiration or hemotogenous from an infected oral focus. May be normal oral flora, especially with decayed teeth.

Predisposing Conditions:

- Tooth Extractions or Eruptions
- Gingivitis
- Diabetes
- Malnutrition
- Immunosupression

CM

Disease manifests as pneumonia, which can be complicated by abscesses, empyema, and pleurodermal sinuses. Cough with purulent sputum, hemoptysis, empyema, chest pain on breathing, clubbing, constitutional symptoms.

CXR

Nonsegmental consolidation, cavitation.

Tx

Antibiotics (high-dose penicillin)

An acute, diffuse, inflammatory lung injury resulting in diminished FRC, severe shunting, alveolar transudates, ↓ surfactant (washout) atelectasis, ↓ compliance, and severe hypoxemia.

ARDS went through a definition clarification in 2013 and is now referred to as the "Berlin definition." Acute lung injury has been replaced by mild, moderate, and severe ARDS.

Diagnostic Criteria:

1. Acute Onset of Respiratory Distress
   Must be within 7 days of a defined event (sepsis, trauma, pneumonia, etc.). Most cases occur within 72 hours.

2. Hypoxemia:

Severity of ARDS	PaO_2/FIO_2 ratio (P/F) (on PEEP ≥ 5 cmH₂O)
Mild	200 - 300
Moderate	100 - 200
Severe	< 100

3. Bilateral consolidation on CXR or CT
   Bilateral infiltrates - diffuse or not (pulmonary edema)

4. Ruled out cardiac failure and fluid overload
   Determined either by PCWP < 18 cmH₂O (noncardiogenic), or by clinical examination (Because PA Catheters are less common, examination techniques, such as echocardiography, are now seen as acceptable)

Phase 1 (first 7-10 days) Exudative
Intense inflammatory response, resulting in:
   • Alveolar and endothelial damage
   • Increased vascular permeability = pulmonary edema
   • Increased water and protein
   • Some component of pulmonary hypertension

Phase 2 (10+ days) Fibroproliferative
Extensive pulmonary fibrosis, which usually resolves
   (acute fibrosis resolves, some fibrosis may remain)

ARDS - Continued Next Page

Respiratory (Direct)	Non-Respiratory (Indirect)
• **Aspiration** (gastric especially) • Near-drowning • O_2 toxicity • Pneumonia (all types) • Post-pneumonectomy • Raised ICP (head injury) • Smoke inhalation • Thoracic irradiation • Severe Thoracic Trauma • Vasculitis	• **Sepsis** (most common cause) • Blood transfusion reactions • Burns (massive) • DIC • Drugs/Alcohol overdose • Fat embolism • Shock (severe, prolonged)

Initial phase is marked by refractory hypoxemia, requiring a high amount of supplemental Oxygen.
After the first few days, the O_2 requirement may decrease.

General	• Agitated, anxious, confused, restless • Rapid-onset (usually within 72 hrs)
Respiratory	• Inspection (cough, cyanosis, dyspnea, retractions, tachypnea, ↑ WOB, diaphoresis) • Palpation (↓ chest expansion) • Auscultation (↓ BS, bronchial BS over consolidation, crackles)
Pulm. Dyn.	• ↓ C_L (total C < 30 mL/cm H_2O) • ↑PIP (vent) • ↓TC; ↑$\dot{V}D$
ABG's	• **Oxygenation** – refractory hypoxemia ($PaO_2/FIO_2 \leq 300$), ↑ shunt (> 20%) • Ventilation – respiratory alkalosis → respiratory acidosis
Cardiovasc.	• ↑ HR • PCWP < 15-18 mm Hg* • PAD – PCWP > 5mmHg

*Compare with CHF: PCWP > 15-18 mm Hg.   (See also Pg 8-12)

ARDS - Continued Next Page

CXR	**2-24 hrs**: Bilateral opacities (diffuse or not) and interstitial infiltrates (peripheral and dependent zones), air broncho-grams.* **24-48 hrs**: coalesce to produce massive air space consolidation in both lungs. * Compare with CHF: cardiomegaly, perihilar infiltrates, pleural effusion.
EBG	• The ARDS Definition Task Force. Acute Respiratory Distress Syndrome: The Berlin Definition. JAMA 2012.
CC	• See **Oakes' Ventilator Management** and **Oakes' Hemodynamic Monitoring** for detailed information
Tx	**General Considerations:** • The goals are to provide supportive care, prevent further injury (to the lungs and elsewhere), and maintain adequate (not normal) oxygenation. • Supplemental oxygen alone may not help (due to the refractory nature of ARDS), so should be used in conjunction with CPAP/PEEP strategies. Mechanical Ventilation is most often required. • Drugs (Analgesics and Sedation) may increase synchrony with the ventilator and ↓ O_2 consumption. • Hemodynamic monitoring (Central Venous Catheter) • Careful fluid management has been shown to improve outcomes (Goal of CVP < ~4 mm Hg). **Specic ventilator strategies are available in Oakes' Ventilator Management.** • Invasive strategies are preferred to NPPV trials • Low VT with goal of Pplat < 30 cmH$_2$O • Use of high PEEP, Recruitment Maneuvers, may be beneficial.

ALVEOLAR HYPOVENTILATION SYNDROMES

Def	Acute or chronic breathing disorder featuring inadequate alveolar ventilation, causing an increased $PaCO_2$.

	Chest Wall Deformities	Kyphoscoliosis, etc.
	COPD	when FEV1 < 1.0 L or < 35% predicted
	Neuromuscular Disorders	Guillain-Barre Syndrome*, Myasthenia Gravis*, Muscular Dystrophy, ALS
	Obesity Hypoventilation Syndrome	Pickwickian. Gross obesity, may occur with OSA, decreased chemical drive to breathe, Lung wall restriction caused by weight on chest
	Primary (Central) Alveolar Hypoventilation	Central Respiratory Drive impairment (Ondine's Curse)

	*See Specific Diseases for Clinical Manifestations	
	Central Alveolar Hypoventilation:	SaO_2 decreases during sleep because of depressed ventilatory response to hypoxia and hypercapnia.
CM	**Obesity Hypoventilation Syndrome**	• Morbid Obesity • Hypoventilation • Hypersomnolence • Fragmented sleep • Hypercapnia, Hypoxemia • Acidemia (may be compensated) • Polycythemia • Cor Pulmonale • Systemic HTN during sleep

	*See Specific Diseases for Treatment Strategies	
Tx	**Obesity Hypoventilation Syndrome**	• Treat OSA (NPPV) • Encourage weight loss • Use PEEP/CPAP to offset chest wall • Recognize and Tx comorbidities • Consider trach in difficult-to-tx

	ALVEOLAR PROTEINOSIS (PAP) *(SEE ALSO INTERSTITIAL LUNG DISEASE)*
Def	Chronic, diffuse, progressive alveolar and interstitial deposition of phospholipoprotein derived from pulmonary surfactant. Links have been made with impaired macrophage maturation/function

	Two Forms:
	  1. Primary (Idiopathic)
	  2. Secondary
	    • Lung Infections
	    • Hematologic malignancies
	    • Inhalation of dusts (silica, aluminum, insecticides, etc.)
	    • Immune Dysfunction (AIDS, Niemann-Pick, etc.)
	
	Usually occurs in people 20-50 years, though rarely may be present at birth

CM	Asymptomatic to death:
	  • Persistent Cough – mild, nonproductive (or scant)
	  • Progressive DOE
	  • Fine Crackles
	  • Hypoxemia (incl. clubbing)
	  • Fatigue, Malaise
	  • Pleuritic Chest Pain
	  • Constitutional symptoms (affect many diff systems)
	  • Samples via BAL appear milky
	
	Mortality Rates generally < 10 %

CXR	Diffuse, bilateral, feathery, butterfly or "bat's wing" pattern.
Tx	• If asymptomatic or minimally symptomatic, may consider observation with no interventions • Bronchial hygiene and lung lavage with normal saline if a-A gradient > 40 mmHg; Dyspnea/Hypoxemia at rest or on exertion; PaO2 < 65 mmHg on RA • Consideration for Blood Stimulating Factor Treatments • If persistent, consideration for lung transplantation

ASPERGILLOSIS

Def	Variety of fungal infections marked by inflammatory granulomatous lesions and aspergillomas (fungus balls). Usually superimposed on individuals with underlying immunosuppression.
Types	**Allergic bronchopulmonary aspergillosis** (ABPA) – asthmatics allergic to Aspergillosis antigen, may present with eosinophilia. **Fungal ball aspergillosis** – fungal ball in cavities. **Invasive aspergillosis** (rare) – chronic necrotizing pneumonia with abscess formation.
	Aspergillus fumigatus/niger (most common). Spores found in soil, decaying organic matter, or building materials. Maybe normal flora in mouth or sputum. **Route** – inhalation or GI tract.
CM	**Asymptomatic to death** – cough with minimal mucoid sputum, recurrent hemoptysis, fever, recurrent pulmonary infections.
CXR	Highly variable – nodules, lesions, nonsegmental consolidation, abscess formation, fungal balls, air cavities, dilated bronchi.
EBG	Clinical Practice Guidelines of the Infectious Diseases Society of America: Treatment of Aspergillosis
Tx	Depends on type – ranges from bronchial hygiene and anti-fungals to resection. ABPA - oral corticosteroids, azole anti-fungal

ASPIRATION PNEUMONIA / PNEUMONITIS

Def	**Aspiration pneumonia**: lung infection caused by chronic aspiration of colonized oropharyngeal secretions. **Aspiration pneumonitis**: acute lung inflammation following aspiration of gastric contents.

Aspiration of bacteria from oropharynx, GI tract, or ventilator circuit condensate. VAP = ventilator associated pneumonia

Aspiration of food particles and acid (↑severity as pH↓)

Contributing Factors:
- Anesthesia/alcohol/drugs
- Convulsions, CPR
- Depressed mental function
- Inadequate cough mechanism
- Impaired gastric emptying
- Impairment of swallowing mechanism

CM		
	Pneumonia (PNA)	Signs of infection with purulent sputum
	Pneumonitis	Sudden tachypnea and dyspnea, cough, crackles, wheezing, cyanosis, hypoxemia, may progress to respiratory failure. PFTs variable

CXR	Patchy, mottled, segmental consolidation (depending on position when aspirated), atelectasis, abscess.

Tx	• Preventive Measures • Airway Clearance (suction) • Oxygen Therapy • Bronchodilators • Therapeutic Bronchoscopy • Invasive ventilatory support, if severe • Antibiotics if indicated • Steroids

ASTHMA

Def	A heterogeneous disease, usually characterized by chronic airway inflammation that is at least partially reversible. It is defined by the history of respiratory symptoms (wheeze, SOB, chest tightness, cough, etc.) that may vary over time and in intensity, together with variable expiratory airflow limitation.
Types	**Extrinsic** (allergic) asthma: 90% of all asthma; typically develops in childhood **Intrinsic** (non-allergic) asthma: 10% of all asthma; develops after age of 30 to 40

<table>
<tr><td rowspan="2">Etiology</td><td>Inhalation</td><td>
• Genetic?
• Allergens:
  • Animal (dander, urine, etc)
  • Pests (cockroach feces, dust mites)
  • Indoor fungi or outdoor pollen, spores
• Occupational exposure:
  • Dust, gases, fumes, chemicals
• Irritants: Air pollution, odors, sprays, stove fumes, tobacco smoke
</td></tr>
<tr><td>Other Factors</td><td>
• Cold air, exercise
• Emotional stress
• Gastroesophageal reflux, food
• Rhinitis/sinusitis
• Sensitivity to drugs (aspirin, beta-blockers, nonsteroidal anti-inflammatory, sulfites)
• Viral respiratory infections
</td></tr>
</table>

<table>
<tr>
<td rowspan="2">CM</td>
<td>
Agitation/restless
Anxiety
Chest tightness
Cough
Diaphoresis
Dyspnea/SOB
Flaring
</td>
<td>
↑RR, ↑HR
↑TE, ↑WOB
Hyperinflation
Hyperreso-
nanceamazon
Hypoxemia
Pulsus paradoxus
Retractions
</td>
<td>
Wheezing*

Late signs:
↓$PaCO_2$ (initial)* →
  ↑$PaCO_2$ (late)
↓ BS
Cyanosis
</td>
</tr>
<tr>
<td colspan="3">DANGER: Respiratory Distress without wheezing (silent chest), or ABG with normal $PaCO_2$ (pt tiring) may indicate impending Respiratory Failure</td>
</tr>
</table>

CM (cont.)	**Is it Asthma? ***
	see also Asthma-COPD Overlap Syndrome in COPD section
	
	The presence of any of these signs and symptoms should increase the suspicion of asthma:
	• Wheezing (but don't exclude consideration if not present)
	• History of:
	  - Cough, worse at night
	  - Recurrent wheeze, difficult breathing, or chest tightness
	• Symptoms occur or worsen at night, awakening patient
	• Patient also has eczema, hayfever, or family hx of asthma
	• Symptoms occur or worsen in the presence of: (see etiology above)
	• Symptoms respond to anti-asthma therapy
	• Patient's colds "go to the chest" or take more than 10 days to clear
	
	* Adapted from Global Initiative for Asthma (GINA), 2016
	
	PFTs: Obstructive Pattern
	↓FVC,↓FEV & FEV₁%,↓PEF ---- ↑FRC, ↑RV, ↑TLC

CXR	Hyperinflation, ↑bronchial markings, flat diaphragm, ↑rib spaces, more radiolucent, narrow heart shadow.

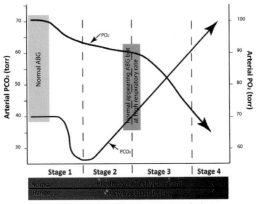

Arterial blood gas, ABG, during various stages of asthma.

11-14

EBG

- Global Strategy for Asthma Management and Prevention - Global Initiative for Asthma (GINA), 2016. Includes a quick reference guide and at-a-glance summaries. ginasthma.org
- International ERS/ATS Guidelines on Definition, Evaluation, and Treatment of Severe Asthma, 2014.

CC

See Oakes Ventilator Management for detailed Mechanical Ventilation strategies related to Asthma

ASTHMA Tx

Levels of Asthma Control*

Characteristic	Controlled (all of the following)	Partly controlled (any measure present in any week)	Uncontrolled
Daytime symptoms	None (≤ 2/week)	> 2/week	
Limitations of Activities	None	Any	
Nocturnal symptoms/ awakening	None	Any	3+ features of partly controlled asthma present in any week
Need for reliever/rescue treatment	None (≤ 2/week)	> 2/week	
Lung Function (PEF or FEV₁)	Normal	< 80% pred or personal best	
Exacerbations	None	≥ 1 /year	1 in any week

* Adapted from Global Initiative for Asthma (GINA). See below.

Asthma Severity, Control, and Treatment

Classifying Severity of Asthma Exacerbations *

Parameter[1]	Mild	Moderate	Severe	Respiratory Arrest Imminent
Breathless	Walking, can lie down	Talking, prefers sitting	At rest, hunched forward	
Talks in	Sentences	Phrases	Words	
Alertness	May be agitated	Usually agitated	Usually agitated	Drowsy or confused
RR[2]	↑	↑	Often > 30/min	
Accessory Muscle Use	None	Usually	Usually	Paradoxical Breathing
Wheeze	Moderate, end-expir	Loud	Usually loud	Absent[ ]
Pulse[3]	<100	100-120	> 120	< 60
Pulsus paradoxus	Absent, < 10mmHg	May be present, 10-25 mmHg	Often present, > 25 mmHg[7]	Absent[7] = respiratory fatigue?
PEF[4]	> 80%	60-80%	< 60% [5]	
PaO2 (on RA)	Normal	> 60mmHg	< 60 mmHg	
PaCO2 [6]	< 45mmHg	< 45 mmHg	> 45 mmHg	
SaO2 (on RA)	> 95%	91-95%	< 90%	

1. The presence of several parameters, but not necessarily all, indicates the general classification of the attack.
2. Normal RR for children: < 2 mo, < 60/min; 2-12 mo, < 50/min; 1-5 yrs, < 40/min; 6-8 yrs, < 30/min.
3. Normal pulse for children: infants (2-12 mo), < 160/min; preschool (1-2 yrs), < 120/min; school age (2-8 yrs), < 110/min.
4. After initial bronchodilator, % pred or % personal best.
5. < 100 L/min adults or response lasts < 2 hrs.
6. Hypercapnia develops more readily in young children than in adults and adolescents.
7. 20-40 mm Hg in children

ASTHMA Tx (continued)

Treatment Strategies See Severity Chart (11-16) for details on Symptoms of Distress	
General Therapy (Mild to Moderate Symptoms)	• Oxygen Therapy should be given to all pts in respiratory distress • Follow oxygenation via SpO_2 or A-Line • Maintain SpO_2 > 90% • Aggressive hydration may be indicated for infants/small children, but is not recommend for older children • CPT, mucolytics, routine CXR, ABG, and sedation are not typically recommended • Inhaled SABA and oral corticosteroids
(Moderate to Severe Symptoms)	• Continuous SABA, ipratropium bromide, and high dose oral or IV steroids • Consider IV Mag sulfate and/or Heliox for pts not responding to initial tx.
Respiratory Failure	• Do not delay Intubation once indicated • Use of NPPV is controversial, but may support pt's ventilatory needs for a short trial. Do not sedate or use in agitated pts. • During BVM, be aware of high risk of air-trapping • May continue Steroids and high-dose bronchodilators when on MV support. • Aim for early extubation post-crisis
Post-Crisis	• Utilize opportunity to do comprehensive education post-crisis. Discussion should include use of an Asthma Plan, Pt demonstration of proper use of medications, as well as indications, etc. • Include family supports as appropriate • Include environmental review (triggers) • Connect pt with Asthma Educator/Program when available. Bilingual services may be available. • Emphasize the controllable nature of Asthma.

ATELECTASIS

Def	Incomplete expansion, non-aeration, and/or collapse of alveoli.

Absorption/Obstructive - absorption of gas from the alveoli after bronchial obstruction (acute: mucous plug, spasm, foreign body; subacute: 100% O_2, retained secretions, tumor).

Compression - compression of lung parenchyma by a space occupying lesion (tumor, pleural effusion, tension pneumothorax).

Hypoventilation - low V_T (anesthesia, drugs, CNS disorder, fatigue, splinting, tight chest dressings, prolonged bed rest, MV)

Micro/Miliary - widespread collapse of alveoli due to loss of or interference with surfactant (e.g., ARDS, O_2 toxicity).

Passive - normal lung retraction when lung is separated from the chest wall (e.g., pneumothorax, pleural effusion).

Post-op - ↓lung expansion (↓ cough and deep breathing)

CM	Asymptomatic to ↑ dyspnea / ↑ WOB ↑ RR / ↑ HR ↓ chest expansion Tracheal shift (same side)	Chest pain, fever, restless Refractory hypoxemia (capillary shunting) **PFTs** – restrictive	**Auscultation over affected area:** late crackles, ↓ BS if airway obstructed, bronchial BS if airway patent, ↑ fremitus, dull percussion note
CXR	Local opacification, air bronchograms, narrowing of rib spaces, elevation of diaphragm on affected side, displacement of heart and trachea towards affected side (unless compression). Micro type = diffuse reticular granular pattern		
Tx	Correct underlying cause. Lung inflation therapy, O_2 therapy, bronchial hygiene, CPAP or MV.		

BACTERIAL PNEUMONIAS

Def

Inflammation of the lungs resulting from a bacterial infection

Types

Atypical: Pneumonia caused by *Mycoplasma*, *Chlamydia* and/or *Legionella*

Bacteriodes species: Anaerobic g-neg rods. Common with bronchiectasis.

Enterobacteria (*Pseudomonas aeruginosa*, *Escherichia coli*, *Proteus species*). Anaerobic g-neg rods. Usually nosocomial, common with bronchiectasis, chronic bronchitis, cystic fibrosis.

Klebsiella pneumoniae: Anaerobic g-neg rods. Similar to pneumococcus, plus necrotizing. Common in diabetic, alcoholic, and chronic lung disease patients.

Haemophilus influenza: Anaerobic, g-neg coccobacilli. Common in COPD.

Legionella pneumophila: Anaerobic, g-neg rod like. Found in contaminated water systems. Causes Legionnaire's disease.

Mycoplasma pneumoniae: viral like organism, community acquired from inhalation of droplet nuclei (use resp. isolation), most common cause of nonbacterial pneumonia (See viral pneumonia)

Serratia marscesens: Anaerobic, g-neg bacilli. May cause pseudohemoptysis, commonly grows in respiratory equipment.

Staphylococcus aureus: Aerobic g-pos cocci. Most common bronchopneumonia (use strict resp. isolation), necrotizing.

Streptococcus pneumoniae: Aerobic g-pos cocci (diplococci). Formerly called pneumococcal pneumonia, 2/3 of all bacterial pneumonia. Often follows URI.

Streptococcus pyogenes: Aerobic g-pos cocci. Usually follows URI, maybe necrotizing.

Etiology

Route: aspiration, inhalation, direct infection via blood.
Predisposing factors: alcoholism, cardiac failure, pre-existing lung disease (asthma, CF, COPD), ↓ cough, debilitation, ET tube, immobility, immuno-compromise, malnutrition, old age, recent smoking, viral respiratory infection.

CM	**May have Rapid Onset of Symptoms, which could be Fatal** • Chills/ Fever • Cough • Cyanosis • Dyspnea / ↑ WOB • Headache/Malaise • ↑RR, ↑HR • Pleural pain • Sputum (See Ch 5) • Tachypnea • Warm, flushed skin • Crackles/ wheeze • Pleural rub (possible) • Bronchial BS/dull percussion over consolidation
CXR	**Lobar** – homogeneous consolidation with well-defined margins. **Bronchial** – patchy, bilateral, peri-bronchial consolidation. **Both** – pleural effusion, cavitation.
EBG	• Infectious Diseases Society of America/American Thoracic Society Consensus Guidelines on the Management of Community-Acquired Pneumonia in Adults • Guidelines for the Management of Adults with Hospital-Acquired, Ventilator-Associated, and Healthcare-Associated Pneumo nia, Official Statement of the American Thoracic Society and the Infectious Diseases Society of America.
Tx	• Antibiotics • Airway Clearance • O₂ therapy. • Pts with more significant infections/manifestations may require Mechanical Ventilation

BLASTOMYCOSIS

Def	Fungal infection initially affecting the lungs, followed by hematogenous dissemination to other organs. Diagnosed via histology
Etiology	*Blastomyces dermatitidis*: inhabits soil, Southeast USA, Mississippi valley, along Great Lakes and St Lawrence river. **Route**: inhalation of spores. Higher Risk: Adults who hunt, fish, camp, operate equipment in high-risk geographical areas
CM	Most acutely infected patients are asymptomatic (or self-limited). Otherwise generally develops into a chronic pneumonia: • Persistent chest pain & tightness, • Dyspnea • Cough • Purulent (bloody or brown) sputum • Low-grade fever • Weight loss • Headache, fatigue, malaise. • May mimic bacterial pneumonia. • Severe cases may develop into ARDS and Resp Failure • Other Systems: • Skin: Lesions with purplish hue around them • Osteoarticular involvement • Prostatitis or epididymitis • Chronic Meningitis (rare)
CXR	Highly variable segmental or lobar consolidation with cavitation. May include pulmonary nodules (cavitating or non)
EBG	• Clinical Practice Guidelines for the Management of Blastomycosis, Infectious Diseases Society of America
Tx	• Systemic Anti-fungal drugs (azoles) • Amphotericin B for severe or life-threatening disease. Once controlled, change to azoles • Airway Clearance, and other Supportive Therapies, as Indicated

BRONCHIECTASIS

Def	Abnormal, permanent dilatation and distortion of one or more conducting airways due to destruction of the elastic and muscular components of the bronchial wall.
Types	**Cylindrical**: Straight tube with abrupt widening **Saccular** (cystic): Outpouchings that balloon outward **Varicose** (fusiform): Gradual widening and tapering
	Acquired bronchiectasis: Necrosis due to frequent or long-standing airway blockage (inhaled foreign object, tumor, or mucus accumulation), infection, immune rx, or noxious chemicals. **Congenital bronchiectasis**: Abnormal airway development.
CM	**Range; Asymptomatic - Death** • Chronic cough – sputum volume varies, maybe mucopurulent, fetid sputum (settles into 3 layers: mucous, saliva, pus) • Hemoptysis / Recurrent infections • DOE • Crackles/wheezes • Clubbing • Hypoxemia leading to cor pulmonale • Weight loss
CXR	Normal to increased bronchovascular markings.
Tx	Prophylaxis, treat infections, control secretions, remove obstructions, treat complications (hemoptysis, hypoxemia, respiratory failure, cor pulmonale), resection?

CARBON MONOXIDE POISONING

Def

Inhalation of CO causing an inhibition of transport, delivery, and utilization of oxygen (decreased SaO_2 & CaO_2, left shift of O_2-Hgb curve, inhibits cytochrome c oxidase).

Auto exhaust, home exhaust, space heaters, obstructed chimney, incomplete combustion of organic materials.

CM

Note: patients do not typically appear "cherry red" and PaO_2 and SpO_2 are usually normal!

Saturation of blood (COHb%)	Symptoms	FICO
0-10%	None	
10-20%	Tightness across forehead, slight headache, dilation of skin vessels.	0.007-0.012
20-30%	Headache, throbbing in temples	0.012-0.022
30-40%	Severe headache, weakness, dizziness, dimness of vision, nausea, vomiting, collapse, syncope, ↑HR, ↑RR.	0.022-0.035
40-50%	Above, plus ↑ tendency to collapse and syncope, ↑HR, ↑RR.	0.035-0.052
50-60%	↑HR, ↑RR, syncope, Cheyne-Stokes respiration, coma with intermittent convulsions.	0.052-0.080
60-70%	Coma with intermittent convulsions, depressed heart action and respiration, death possible.	0.080-0.120
70-80%	Weak pulse, depressed respiration, respiratory failure, death.	0.120-0.195

These are general guidelines. Some patients may be asymptomatic until COHb% > 40%

Clinical symptoms and COHb levels often do not coincide –
Treat whichever is the most severe.

> 10% COHb, w/ headache, or blurred vision:	Give 100% oxygen. Use tight fitting non-rebreather mask, ET tube, or other. Continue until < 10 %.
> 15% COHb:	100% O_2, plus admit to hospital if history of heart disease.
> 25% COHb abnormal neuro or CV exam, unconscious, severe acidosis, pregnant woman, or age > 60:	Give 100% O_2, plus transport to hyperbaric chamber is highly recommended.

Half-Life of COHb

In Air	300 minutes
In 100% O_2	90 minutes
@ 2.5 ATA (hyperbarics)	30 minutes

- Monitor Cardiac, ABG's and COhb level
- Intubate and ventilate if unconscious or uncooperative
- Avoid hyperventilation and $NaHCO_3$ (shifts oxy-heme curve to left)
- Steroids or hypothermia?
- Watch for latent deterioration (usually 4-9 days later), pulmonary edema, MI, CHF. Hyperbaric oxygenation (HBO) within 24 hrs of hospitalization reduces the risk for cognitive sequelae compared with standard normobaric O_2 therapy.

	CARDIAC TAMPONADE
Def	Acute, abnormal accumulation of fluid in pericardial sac resulting in heart compression.
Etiology	Hemorrhage (aneurysm, rupture, trauma) or pericarditis (infection, MI, surgery).
CM	Proportional to degree of heart compression (asymptomatic to total CV collapse), pulsus paradoxus, sinus tachycardia, Beck's triad (JVD [or ↓CVP], ↓BP, muffled heart).
CXR	Cardiac enlargement (water bottle shape), clear lungs
CC	See Oakes' Hemodynamic Monitoring for comprehensive information on Cardiac Tamponade
Tx	• Immediate pericardiocentesis • Maintain adequate CO • O₂ therapy as needed • Pericardiectomy?

	CHRONIC BRONCHITIS
Def	**Bronchitis** - inflammation of bronchial mucosa due to infection or chemical inhalation. **Chronic** - cough with excessive mucus production occurring on most days for at least three consecutive months for 2 years in a row. **Chronic bronchitis** – diagnosis based on symptomatology; a principal manifestation of COPD.
Etiology	Chronic irritation (smoking, air pollution), infections (viral, bacterial), hereditary.
CM	See COPD for Clinical Manifestations, CXR, Evidence-Based Guidelines, and Treatment Strategies

CHRONIC OBSTRUCTIVE PULMONARY DISEASE (COPD)

Def

A preventable and treatable disease that is characterized by persistent airflow limitation that is usually progressive. It is associated with chronic inflammatory responses in the airways and the lungs to noxious particles or gases.

Asthma is not classified as COPD.

Asthma-COPD Overlap Syndrome: *Persistant airflow limitation with several features usually associated with both asthma and COPD.*

- The chronic airflow limitation characteristic of COPD is caused by a mixture of small airway disease (obstructive bronchiolitis) and parenchymal destruction (emphysema), the relative contributions of which vary from person to person.

Diagnosis:
- A diagnosis of COPD should be considered in any pt who has dyspnea (persistent and progressive), chronic cough, or sputum production and/or a history of exposure to risk factors, especially cigarette smoking, occupational dusts and chemicals, and/or indoor/outdoor pollution.
- The diagnosis should be confirmed by spirometry (FEV_1, FVC, FEV_1/FVC ratio < 70%)
- There may be a genetic component to COPD: Alpha-1 Antitrypsin Disorder (Alpha-1). The ATS, AARC, and ACCP all recommend routine, blood-based testing for Alpha-1 in all patients with suspected COPD.
- Research shows the greater the number of comorbidities, the more severe the Dyspnea in patients with COPD.

EBG
- ACCP, ATS, ERS
- GOLD
- Cochrane Reviews
- ICSI

CC
- See Oakes' Hemodynamic Monitoring for detailed Cardio-pulmonary Function
- See Oakes' Ventilator Management for detailed Mechanical Ventilation Strategies

Comparison of Clinical Manifestations*

Characteristic	Emphysema (Pink Puffer)	Chronic Bronchitis (Blue Bloater)
Inspection		
Body	thin	stocky or fat (bloater)
Chest	barrel chest	normal
	hypertrophy of accessory muscles	↑ use of accessory muscles
Breathing Pattern	progressive dyspnea	variable
	labored (puffer)	normal
	retractions	normal
	↓ chest movement	normal
	↓ IE ratio, ↑ T_E	↑IE ratio, ↓ T_E
Posture	orthopnea	varibale
Cough	slight	considerable
Sputum	small amt - mucoid	large amt - purulent
Color	normal (pink)	cyanosis (blue)
Palpation	norm to ↓ fremitus	norm to ↓ fremitus
Auscultation		
BS	↓	norm to ↓
Wheezing	slight	episodic
Blood Gases		
PaO_2 resting	Slight ↓	Mod to Severe ↓
PaO_2 exercise	falls	stable
$PaCO_2$	norm	↑
HCO_3	norm	↑
PFT's**		
Spirometry	obstructive	obstructive
RV and TLC	↑	norm to ↓
Diffusion Capacity	↓	normal
Compliance	↑	normal
Hematocrit	< 55%	> 55%
ECG	right axis deviation	RVH
CXR		
Broncho-vascular markings	↓	↑
Hyperinflation	yes	no
Bullae/blebs	yes	no
Past History	normal	freq resp infections
Lifespan	norm (60-80 yrs)	shorter (40-60 yrs)
Cor pulmonale	uncommon	common
Death	nonpulmonary or RF	RVF or RF

Notes from Previous Page

See also Pg 1-16, 8-12 and Oakes' *Hemodynamic Monitoring: A Bedside Reference Manual* for greater detail.

* Pure chronic bronchitis or emphysema is rarely seen. Most commonly it is a combination of both.

** The diagnosis of COPD is confirmed by spirometry: the presence of a post-bronchodilator $FEV_1 < 80\%$ predicted, plus an $FEV_1/FVC < 70\%$.

The following section is a brief summary of the Global Strategy for the Diagnosis, Management and Prevention of COPD, Global Initiative for Chronic Obstructive Lung Disease (GOLD) 2016. Available from: http://www.goldcopd.org.

Stages of COPD

Severity	Symptoms	Spirometry	Treatment
Stage I: Mild	Chronic cough and sputum (maybe)	$FEV_1/FVC < 70\%$ $FEV_1 \geq 80\%$ predicted	Avoid risk factors Obtain flu vaccine SABA prn
Stage II: Moderate	Progression of above, + DOE	$FEV_1/FVC < 70\%$ FEV_1 50% to 79% predicted	Above, and: Scheduled LABA Pulm. Rehab
Stage III: Severe	↑ SOB + repeated exacerbations	$FEV_1/FVC < 70\%$ FEV_1 30% to 49% predicted	Above, and: ICS if repeated exacerbations
Stage IV: Very Severe	Impaired quality of life and exacerbations may be life-threatening	$FEV_1/FVC < 70\%$ FEV_1 <30% pred or < 50%, plus chronic resp. failure or RHF	Above, and: Long-term O_2 therapy if chronic resp. failure Consider surgical options

Key:
SABA: Short-Acting Beta Agonist; LABA: Long-Acting Beta Agonist
ICS: Inhaled Corticosteroid. See PFT chapter for details on spirometry tests.

The Four Components of COPD Management

1. Assess and Monitor
2. Reduce Risk Factors
3. Manage Stable COPD
4. Manage Exacerbations

1. Assess and Monitor

- Detailed medical history
- ABG's (see below)
- Bronchodilator reversibility test
- CXR
- Spirometry
- Alpha-1 antitrypsin deficiency screen (family Hx or < 45 yrs)

2. Reduce Risk Factors

Smoking cessation, minimize occupational exposures and indoor/outdoor pollutions.

3. Managing Stable COPD

Do's:

ABGs should be considered for patients with FEV1 < 50 % predicted or signs of respiratory failure (central cyanosis, PaO_2 < 60 mm Hg +/or SaO_2 < 90% (room air) with or without $PaCO_2$ > 50 mm Hg) or RHF (ankle swelling and ↑ JV pressure).

Bronchodilator drugs: (central to symptom management)
- β2-agonists, anticholinergics, and methylxanthines – choice depends on availability and patient's response.
- Inhaled therapy is preferred
- Long-acting inhaled are more effective and convenient.
- Combining bronchodilators may improve efficacy and ↓ side effects compared to ↑ dose of a single bronchodilator.
- Wet nebulizers may provide subjective benefit in acute episodes.
- In general, nebulized therapy for a stable patient is not appropriate unless shown to be better than conventional dose therapy.

Inhaled glucocorticosteroids may reduce the risk of repeated hospitalizations and death. They should be considered for patients with an FEV_1 < 50% , repeated exacerbations requiring oral steroids, and/or objective evidence of response to a trial of inhaled corticosteroids.

O_2 therapy: Keep PaO_2 at least 60 mm Hg and/or SaO_2 at least 90% (at rest).

Long-term O_2 therapy (> 15 hrs/day) is generally introduced at Stage IV in patients with: 1) PaO_2 ≤ 55 mm Hg or SaO_2 ≤ 88% on room air, with or without hypercapnia.; or 2) PaO_2 55 - 60 mm Hg or SaO_2 ≤ 88% on room air, if there is evidence of pulmonary hypertension, peripheral edema (CHF), or hematocrit > 55%.

Patient education: Smoking cessation (The 5 As –See Ch 12), etc.

Systemic steroids are clinically beneficial to patients hospitalized with an exacerbation. (Chronic therapy should be avoided).

Don'ts:

Antibiotics, other than for treating infectious exacerbations, are not recommended.

Antitussives: regular use is not recommended.

Mast cell stabilizers or leukotriene modifiers are not recommended.

Mucolytic agents are generally not recommended.

N-acetylcysteine (antioxidant) may or may not have a role in treating exacerbations.

Nitric oxide is contraindicated.

4) Managing Exacerbations

Diagnosis of an Exacerbation

↑ breathlessness, often accompanied by wheezing and chest tightness ↑ cough and purulent sputum (altered color +/or tenacity), and fever.	Also may present with ↑RR, ↑HR, malaise, insomnia, fatigue, depression, and confusion.

Note: The most important sign of severe exacerbation is a change in mental status

Assessing Severity of an Exacerbation

ABGs:

- Respiratory failure = room air $PaO_2 < 60$ mm Hg, &/or $SaO_2 < 90\%$ with or without $PaCO_2 > 50$ mm Hg
- Mechanical ventilation is indicated when pH < 7.36, $PaCO_2 > 45-60$ mm Hg, and $PaO_2 < 60$ mm Hg.

Chest x-ray: identify complications/alternative diagnoses mimicking an exacerbation.

ECG: helps identify RV hypertrophy, arhythmias, and ischemic episodes.

Note: Low BP and inability to ↑ PaO_2 may suggest pulmonary embolism

Spirometry: is not recommended

Management

Indications for ICU Admission:

- Severe unresponsive dyspnea, confusion, lethargy, coma
- Life threatening ABGs (severe or worsening $PaO_2 < 40$ mm Hg, and/or $PaCO_2 > 60$ mm Hg, and/or pH < 7.25, despite O_2 and NIPPV therapy)
- Invasive MV and/or
- Hemodynamic instability (vasopressors needed).

Bronchodilator therapy: Short-acting, inhaled B2-agonists are preferred. If prompt response does not occur, then anticholinergics recommended. Role of aminophylline is controversial.

Glucocorticosteroids: Oral or intravenous are recommended as an addition to bronchodilator therapy.

O_2 Therapy: Maintain $PaO_2 > 60$ mm Hg, SaO_2 88-92%. Check 30 min after initiating O_2 therapy.

CPT and PD: Not recommended unless co-existing bronchiectasis

Antibiotics: Give –

- With ↑ dyspnea, sputum volume and/or purulence
- When MV is required

Respiratory stimulants (doxapram) are not recommended.

Ventilation: See Oakes' ***Ventilator Management: A Bedside Reference Guide*** for indications and a detailed discussion.

Management of Severe but Not Life-Threatening Exacerbations of COPD in the Emergency Department or the Hospital

- Assess severity of symptoms, ABGs, CXR
- Administer controlled O_2 therapy and repeat ABG after 30-60 min
- Bronchodilators:
  - Increase doses or frequency
  - Combine β2-agonists and anticholinergics
  - Use spacers or air-driven nebulizers
  - Add IV methylxanthine, if needed
- Add glucocorticosteroids — Oral or intravenous.
- Consider antibiotics with signs of bacterial infection (↑ in dyspnea, sputum volume, purulence)
  - oral or occasionally intravenous
- Consider NPPV. There is some concern with extended mechanical ventilation (invasive in particular) that atrophy of accessory muscles (critical in how severe COPDers maintain acceptable ventilation/oxygenation) may occur, making weaning a difficult, if not impossible, task.
- At all times:
  - Monitor fluid balance and nutrition
  - Consider subcutaneous heparin
  - Identify/treat associated conditions (e.g., heart failure, arrhythmias)
  - Closely monitor condition of the patient

See:

Global Strategy for the Diagnosis, Management and Prevention of COPD, 2016 Update, Global Initiative for Chronic Obstructive Lung Disease (GOLD). Available from: www.goldcopd.org.

Also, see Oakes' **Ventilator Management: A Bedside Reference Guide** for further details and strategies for mechanical ventilation of the COPD patient.

COPD Indications for Noninvasive and Invasive Ventilation

See <u>Oakes' Ventilator Management</u> for detailed COPD ventilatory strategies

Indications for Noninasive Mechanical Ventilation[1]

At least one of the following:

- Respiratory Acidosis (art. pH ≤ 7.35 and/or $PaCO_2$ ≥ 45 mm Hg)
- Severe dyspnea with clinical signs suggestive of respiratory muscle fatigue, increased WOB, or both, such as:
  - use of respiratory accessory muscles
  - paradoxical motion of the abdomen, or
  - retraction of the intercostal spaces

Indications for Invasive Mechanical Ventilation[1]

- Unable to tolerate NIV or NIV failure
- Respiratory or cardiac arrest
- Respiratory pauses with loss of consciousness, or gasping for air
- Diminished consciousness, psychomotor agitation inadequately controlled by sedation
- Massive aspiration
- Persisitent inability to remove respiratory secretions
- Heart rate < 50/min with loss of alertness
- Severe hemodynamic instability without response to fluids and vasoactive drugs
- Severe ventricular arrhythmias
- Life-threatening hypoxemia in patients unable to tolerate NIV

---

[1] Adapted from Global Strategy for the Diagnosis, Management, and Prevention of COPD, 2016 Update

CLUBBING
(HYPERTROPHIC PULMONARY OSTEOARTHROPATHY)

Def

A syndrome of bulbous enlargement of the terminal phalanges, arthritis, and periostitis due to overgrowth and inflammatory changes in the soft tissue.

Primary cause unknown: Theories – hypoxia of local tissues, capillary stasis, chronic infections, A-V shunts.

Pulmonary: Alveolar proteinosis, chronic hypoxemia, pneumoconiosis, pulmonary infections, empyema, tumors, UIP.

Nonpulmonary: Bacterial endocarditis, CHD, hereditary, liver cirrhosis, long-term MV.

Unilateral clubbing: Local or aortic aneurysms, pulmonary hypertension with PDA..

CM

Skin-nail angle > 160°

Normal	Early	Advanced
< 160°	< 180°	< 200°

COCCIDIOIDOMYCOSIS

Def	Systemic fungal infection characterized by caseating granulomas and its prevalence in the southwest USA.
Etiology	*Coccidioides immitis*, inhabits soil in semi arid regions. Most common source: dust storms, farming. **Route**: inhalation.
CM	Asymptomatic (majority) to death -- • Poorly localized chest pain aggravated by breathing • Nonproductive cough • Hemoptysis • Constitutional (other systems) symptoms. • Meningitis is common cause of death.
CXR	Nodules, cavitation, bronchopneumonia, hilar enlargement, pleural effusion.
Tx	• Anti-fungal drugs (amphotericin B) - severe cases • Various azoles • Airway Clearance • Surgical for severe hemoptysis • BP fistula or persistent cavitary growth

DISEASES

See Oakes' Ventilator Management and Oakes' Hemodynamic Monitoring for Critical Care Considerations for all relevant Diseases and Disorders

Oakes' Ventilator Management
An Oakes Pocket Guide

Dana Oakes
Sean Shortall
Scot Jones

CONGESTIVE HEART FAILURE (LEFT HEART FAILURE, LVF)

Def	Inability of the left ventricle to maintain adeq. CO, thereby failing to provide sufficient blood flow to meet the metabolic demands of the body. Usually LHF with/without RHF.
Etiology	Many and various – Arrhythmias, acquired or congenital HD, infection, ischemia, shock.
CM	**Cardiac:** ↑HR, murmurs (S3), ↓BP, peripheral edema, JVD, hepatomegaly **Respiratory:** ↑RR, dyspnea, othopnea, crackles/wheeze, hypoxemia, cough (pink, frothy), PND, pulsus alternans. **Other:** Fatigue, irritable, sweating
CXR	Cardiomegaly, ↑pulmonary vasculature? Kerly B lines
EBG	• ACC/AHA Guideline Update for the Diagnosis and Management of Chronic Heart Failure in the Adult • Chronic Heart Failure: Management of chronic heart failure in adults in primary and secondary care (NICE) • 2010 Heart Failure Society of America Comprehensive Heart Failure Practice Guideline
CC	• See Oakes' Hemodynamic Monitoring for detailed Cardiopulmonary Function • See Oakes' Ventilator Management for detailed Mechanical Ventilation Strategies
Tx	• Treat cause and complications (pulmonary edema) • O₂ therapy • ↑CO (↓afterload, adequate preload, ↑ myocardial contractility, prevent dysrhythmias) • Keep HOB > 10-45 degrees • Consider NPPV with adequate EPAP • Mechanical Ventilation with adequate PEEP to decrease WOB, unload LV • Restrict Intake, Diurese • Correct anemia and electrolytes

SEE ALSO Pulmonary Edema

COR PULMONALE (RT HEART FAILURE, RHF)

Def	RV hypertrophy and dilatation caused by pulmonary disease
Etiology	**Pulmonary hypertension due to:** **Anatomical increase:** Vascular disease, diffuse interstitial fibrosis, granulomas, emphysema. **Vascular motor increase:** Hypoxemia, hypercarbia, acidosis. **Combined:** Multiple small pulmonary emboli. ↑ blood flow, volume, or viscosity (polycythemia). **Note:** Neither LHD nor CHD is included as a factor. **Acute cor pulmonale:** pulmonary embolism & ARDS.
CM	• Dyspnea • Cough • Chest discomfort • Hepatomegaly • Peripheral edema • JVD • Hypoxemia • Cyanosis • ↓$PaCO_2$ • ↑ Hematocrit • ECG Δ.
CXR	Right ventricular enlargement
CC	• See **Oakes' Hemodynamic Monitoring** for detailed Cardio-pulmonary Function • See **Oakes' Ventilator Management** for detailed Mechanical Ventilation Strategies
Tx	• Tx underlying lung disease • Reduce RV afterload • Relieve cause of pulmonary hypertension • O_2 therapy • Diuretics, calcium channel blockers, anticoagulants to reduce risk of blood clots

CRYPTOCOCCOSIS

Def	Pulmonary fungal infection that can disseminate throughout the body
	Inhalation of *Cryptococcus neoformans* (G+ yeast) spores. Inhabits soil rich in pigeon droppings.
CM	Varies from asymptomatic (most common) to ARDS: • Cough with mucoid sputum • Hemoptysis • Pleuritic pain, • Dyspnea • Fever.
CXR	Multiple nodules or diffuse infiltrates, bronchopneumonia, occasional cavitation.
EBG	• Clinical Practice Guidelines for the Management of Cryptococcal Disease, 2010 Update by the Infectious Disease Society of America
Tx	Amphotericin B with/without flucytosine for several weeks, afterward oral fluconazole

CUSHING'S SYNDROME

Def	Clinical syndrome characterized by the manifestations listed below.
	↑ Corticosteroids either by adrenal gland production or chronic iatrogenic administration.
CM	Fat deposition: moon face, buffalo hump, truncal obesity. Muscle weakness and fatigability, osteoporosis, diabetic mellitus, hypertension, emotional changes.

DIABETIC KETOACIDOSIS (DKA)

Def

Metabolic acidosis caused by accumulation of ketone bodies from tissue protein breakdown.

Respiratory Involvement: Significant Metabolic Acidosis will result in Respiratory Compensation (hyperventilation), with eventual tiring resulting in Respiratory Failure and a combined, sometimes significant Mixed Acidosis.

Criteria

- Insufficient insulin in known diabetes (or undiagnosed)
- Diagnostic Criteria (2009 ADA)

	Mild	Moderate	Severe
Plasma Glucose > 250 mg/dL			
Arterial pH	7.25 - 7.30	7.00-7.24	< 7.00
Serum HCO_3	15-18	10-14	< 10
Ketones (serum/urine)	+	+	+
Anion Gap	> 10	> 12	> 12
Mental Status	Alert	Drowsy	Stupor/ Coma
$PaCO_2$	Alkalosis	Alkalosis or Normal	Acidosis

CM

- Kussmaul breathing ($\downarrow PaCO_2$),
- Sweet breath odor (ketones)
- Vomiting, Headache, Dehydration
- $\downarrow$ Na+, $\downarrow$ K+,
- Coma, Long-Term Neurological disruption

EBG

- American Diabetes Association: Standards of Medical Care in Diabetes

Tx

- Correct acidosis (bicarb if < 6.90)
- Fluid Infusions with careful consideration of electrolytes
- Careful glucose/insulin control and monitoring (give insulin once K+ deficiencies have been corrected. Administration of bicarb may further complicate K+ control)
- Support Respiratory status, as required

EMPHYSEMA

Def	Enlargement and destruction of the air spaces beyond the terminal bronchiole.
Types	**Panlobular**: Affects alveoli, alveolar ducts and sacs **Alpha-1 Antitrypsin Deficiency** **Centribolular**: Affects respiratory bronchioles
Etiology	**Panlobular**: constitutional defect, idiopathic, alpha-1 anti-trypsin (genetic) deficiency generally manifesting by the 4th to 5th decade **Centribolular**: Smoking, air pollution, chronic bronchitis, infection, occupational exposure to dusts
CM	See COPD
CXR	See COPD
EBG	• See *ATS/ERS Statement: Standards for the Diagnosis and Management of Individuals with Alpha-1 Antitrypsin Deficiency*
CC	• See Oakes' *Ventilator Management for Mechanical Ventilation Strategies*
Tx	See COPD

Figure contents (Types):

Normal	Centrilobular	Panlobular
terminal bronchiole, resp. bronchiole		

EMPYEMA

Def	Purulent fluid in the pleural cavity.
Etiol	Extension of infection from pneumonia, lung abscess, sub-diaph. abscess, pneumothorax, trauma, bronchiectasis, TB
CM	Signs and symptoms of the infection, plus physical signs of fluid in the pleural cavity. See pleural effusion.
CXR	Fluid in the pleural space and or pleural thickening.
Tx	Chest tube drainage or surgery

FLAIL CHEST

Def	Condition in which a portion of the chest wall moves in a direction opposite to the rest of the thorax. Instability due to fractures of two or more ribs in at least two locations.
Etiol	Chest trauma (usually mechanical such as in automobile crashes and industrial machinery accidents)
CM	Paradoxical movement of chest wall. Reduced ventilation to affected side, dyspnea, ↑WOB, pain, splinting, atelectasis, hypoxemia. Usually accompanied by other pulmonary injuries.
CXR	Fractured ribs
CC	• See **Oakes' Ventilator Management** for Mechanical Ventilation Strategies
Tx	• Airway Clearance Therapies • Pain management to encourage deep breathing • If chest needs to be stabilized, use external fixation and Mechanical Ventilation (PEEP?)

GUILLAIN-BARRÉ SYNDROME (GBS)

Def	A heterogenous syndrome that causes (usually) ascending muscular paralysis following an infection
	Most have neurological symptoms 2-4 weeks after febrile resp or GI infection. Note that there are multiple subtypes (AIDP, AMAN, AMSAN, MFS, etc.)
CM	**Progressive, Mostly Symmetric Symptoms:** • Ascending muscle weakness/↓ reflexes (may vary) • Lumbar Puncture: ↑ CSF protein with normal CSF WBC • EMG: acute denervation is a serious sign for prognosis
CC	See **Oakes' Ventilator Management** for strategies
Tx	Closely monitor pulmonary mechanics and airway control. Bronchial hygiene, & lung expansion to ↓ atelectasis, intubation/MV at VC ≈20 mL/kg and/or poor upper airway control. Plasmaphoresis, high dose immune globulin therapy?

HISTOPLASMOSIS

Def	Chronic systemic fungal infection characterized by prevalence in East Central USA and Mississippi Valley.
	Histoplasma capsulatum, inhabits soil rich with pigeon, bird, chicken, and bat droppings. **Route**: inhalation.
CM	Asymptomatic (majority) to fatal. Respiratory tract infection of varying severity. Dyspnea, chest pain, crackles, cough with scant mucoid sputum, constitutional symptoms.
CXR	Highly variable, cavitation, hilar calcification, widespread infiltrates.
EBG	**Clinical Practice Guidelines for the Management of Patients with Histoplasmosis, Update by the Infectious Diseases Society of America**
Tx	Anti-fungal drugs if moderate or severe.

HYPERSENSITIVITIY PNEUMONIA (ALLERGIC ALVEOLITIS)

Def	Extrinsic allergic pneumonias occurring in workers sensitized to organic dusts.
Types	Bagassosis, bird-breeder's lung, farmer's lung, humidifier lung, etc.
Etiology	Organic dusts (bacteria, fungi, animal proteins, chemicals).
CM	Depends on antigen type, concentration, size, shape, patient sensitivity, length of time/amount of exposure. Dyspnea, cough, chest tightness, wheezing/crackles, tachypnea, hypoxemia, PFT's – restrictive, constitutional symptoms.
CXR	Varies with specific etiology. ↑ bronchovascular markings, diffuse finely modular shadows, hyperinflation, honeycombing.
Tx	Avoid antigens, treat symptoms, steroids for acute forms.

INFLUENZA

Def	Acute respiratory tract viral infection characterized by the sudden onset of symptoms.
Etiology	Viral: influenza A, B, C
CM	Sudden onset of constitutional symptoms, plus rhinitis, pharyngitis, tracheitis, bronchitis, pneumonia. Range of severity varies from minimally symptomatic to life-threatening.
Tx	Because this is viral, only limited options are available (which slow the progression, decreasing severity and length of the illness). Respiratory goals are to provide supportive care (support ventilation, oxygenation, etc., as indicated by clinical presentation)

INTERSTITIAL LUNG DISEASE (ILD)
INTERSTITIAL PNEUMONIA

Def	A large variety (150) of diffuse pulmonary infiltrative disorders characterized by alveolar wall injury leading to the development of interstitial / alveolar exudates, hyaline membranes, and fibrosis.
Etiology	• Idiopathic pulmonary fibrosis (50%) • (Alveolar proteinosis, BOOP, DIP, Hamman-Rich, Sarcoidosis, ,UIP) • Chemical irritants • Collagen disorder's (Goodpastures, SLE) • Drug-induced (illicit or medications, O_2 toxicity, radiation therapy) • Familial disorders • Infections • Neoplasms • Prolonged circulatory failure • Occupational lung disease (See Hypersensitivity pneumonia, Pneumoconiosis)
CM	**Varies with extent of involvement:** • DOE (most common) • Cough (maybe productive) • Crackles • Clubbing/Fatigue • Hypoxemia leading to cor pulmonale • Respiratory alkalosis • PFTs-restrictive • Constitutional sympt.
CXR	Varies with stage, normal or reticulonodular densities or ground glass haziness and honeycombing
EBG	**The Official Statement of the ATS/ERS/JRS/ALAT: Idiopathic Pulmonary Fibrosis: Evidence-based Guidelelines for Diagnosis and Management**
Tx	Avoid exposure, O_2 therapy?, steroids?, cytotoxic agents?

SEE ALSO Hypersensitivity Pneumonia (Organic), Pneumoconiosis (Inorganic), and Sarcoidosis

11-44

KYPHOSCOLIOSIS

Def	Angulation of the vertebral column resulting in a restrictive chest wall disorder. **Kyphosis**: posterior curvature of the spine **Scoliosis**: lateral curvature of the spine
Etiology	Idiopathic (80%), congenital, bone Tuberculsosi, neuromuscular disorder.
CM	Marked chest asymmetry, marked variations in chest excursion and BS, DOE, ↓ Ccw, ↑ WOB, ↑ $PaCO_2$, hypoxemia leading to cor pulmonale, polycythemia, atelectasis, recurrent pulmonary infections, PFT's – restrictive.
CXR	Marked bone deformation, atelectasis..
CC	See **Oakes' Ventilator Management** for Mechanical Ventilation Strategies
Tx	Spinal fixation, lung inflation therapy, bronchial hygiene.

LUNG ABSCESS

Def	Inflammatory necrotic lesion of the lung parenchyma that contains purulent material.
Etiology	Aspiration of oro/nasopharyngeal contents containing necrotic infectious organisms (usually anaerobes).
CM	Highly variable. Most common: periodic cough with expectoration of large amounts of purulent, fetid, bloody sputum. Dull chest pain, consolidation (dull to percussion), crackles, clubbing, ↓ BS, (maybe cavernous), constitutional symptoms.
CXR	Definitive diagnosis: rounded area of dense infiltration surrounding a radiolucent center which may present with a horizontal air-fluid interface.
Tx	Antibiotics, postural drainage.

LUNG CANCERS (LUNG CA)

Def	A disease of uncontrolled cell growth in tissues of the lung, which may lead to metastasis beyond the lungs.
Types	Non-small cell lung cancer (NSCLC): 85%, adenocarcinoma (most common), squamous (epithelial) cell, large cell undifferentiated Small-cell lung cancer (SCLC), or Oat Cell Carcinoma: 15%, most aggressive
Etiology	**Primary cause:** 85% linked to smoking (COPD) **Secondary causes:** hereditary, racial, dietary, occupational/environmental exposure (air pollution, asbestos, radiation, radon).

CM

Asymptomatic to death, depending on type/stage of cancer. Stage is the extent the cancer has spread (metastasis and degree of lung involvement).

Persistent cough Chest pain/dyspnea	Hemoptysis Localized wheezing	Repeated infections Clubbing

Staging

IA: T1N0M0 IB: T2N0M0	IIA: T1N1M0 IIB: T2N1M0 T3N0M0	IIIA: T3N1M0 T(1-3)N2M0 IIIB: T4N(0-3)M0 T(1-4)N3M0	IV: T(any) N(any)M1

CXR	Atelectasis, rounded masses of variable size and shape, unilateral hilar enlargement, consolidation, pleural effusion. CAT and PET Scans provide type & location details
EBG	**Diagnosis and Management of Lung Cancer Executive Summary: ACCP Evidence-Based Clinical Practice Guidelines**
Tx	**Bronchoalveolar involvement:** smoking cessation therapy, O₂ therapy, lung inflation therapy, Airway Clearance Therapy, pulm rehab. **NSCLC:** Surgical resection is treatment of choice for early stage, chemotherapy for advanced stage **SCLC:** Chemotherapy with or without radiotherapy

MYOCARDIAL INFARCTION (MI)
ACUTE CORONARY SYNDROME (ACS)

Def	Acute myocardial ischemia → necrosis of cardiac muscle
Types	Acute ST Elevation MI (STEMI) Non-ST Elevation MI (N-STEMI) Unstable Angina (UA)
Etiology	↓ coronary artery perfusion resulting from coronary artery disease (atherosclerosis) or spasm; ventricular hypertrophy; hypoxia
CM	Dependent on location and extent of ischemic damage and resultant myocardial damage. Common findings: ↑ HR, chest pain (angina pectoris) /radiating pain (teeth, jaw, neck, shoulder, ↓ arm), SOB, orthopnea, nausea, diaphoresis, anxiety.
CC	• See Oakes' *Hemodynamic Monitoring* for greater details • See Oakes' *Ventilator Management* for Mechanical Ventilation Strategies
Tx	• Stabilize airway and breathing • O₂ Therapy SaO₂ < 90%, respiratory distress, heart failure, or other high-risk features for hypoxia (maintain > 90%) • O₂ for normoxic (> 94%) pts is controversial - may be harmful, having a direct vasoconstrictive effect on coronary arteries • Stabilize hemodynamic status (maintain optimal CO/ tissue perfusion) • Reduce Ischemia (coronary re-perfusion: primary percutaneous coronary intervention [PCI], fibrinolysis, coronary artery bypass graft [CABG]) • Drugs (anti-platelet [aspirin], anticoagulants [heparin], anti-dysrhythmics, β-blockers, nitrates, morphine, ACE inhibitors, statin therapy) • Therapy and management depends on type, timing, severity • NPPV, if needed

MYASTHENIA GRAVIS

Def	Disorder of neuromuscular transmission of the voluntary (skeletal) muscles characterized by muscle weakness and easy fatigability, which often affects the respiratory muscles.
Etiology	Acquired auto-immune disorder. Note: A "myasthenic syndrome" sometimes accompanies sarcoidosis, hyper or hypothyroidism and lung cancer.
CM	Extreme weakness and fatigability, choking, aspiration, respiratory insufficiency. Diagnosed and temporary relief by anti-cholinesterase drugs (neostigmine bromide, edrophonium). Typical presentation is **descending** symptoms. **Myasthenic crisis**: acute event characterized by respiratory compromise. **Cholinergic crisis**: over-treatment of anti-cholinesterase (clinical presentation similar to a myasthenic crisis). **Note**: Tensilon test: Give edrophonium chloride – if myasthenic crisis, pt improves; if cholinergic crisis, pt worsens.
CC	• See **Oakes' Ventilator Management** for Mechanical Ventilation Strategies
EBG	International Consensus Guidance for Management of MG
Tx	Monitor pulmonary mechanics and airway control, anti-cholinesterase (pyridostigmine) drugs, bronchial hygiene, Mech Vent, immunomodulating agents, steroids?, Plasmaphoresis?, immune globulin?, thymectomy?

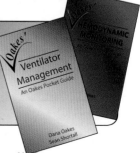

See **Oakes' Ventilator Management** and **Oakes' Hemodynamic Monitoring** for Critical Care Considerations for all relevant Diseases and Disorders

	NEAR-DROWNING (DROWNING)
Def	A process resulting in primary respiratory impairment from submersion/immersion in liquid. The victim may live (survival) or die (death by drowning) after this process. Although still used, the term *near drowning* is no longer recommended.
Types	Differences between fresh and salt water near drowning are clinically unimportant. Water temperature and the presence of contaminants in the water are greater considerations than the salinity.
Etiology	Leaving small children unattended, trauma (head/neck), exhaustion, intoxication (alcohol, drugs), seizures.
CM	Variable with minimal findings to cardiorespiratory arrest (often a delay of 2-6 hrs). **Pulmonary**: hypoxemia, SOB, tachypnea, cyanosis, pallor, crackles, frothy sputum, wheezing, cough, apnea. **Cerebral**: changed mental status, seizures, stupor, coma. **Other**: arrhythmias, evidence of trauma, metabolic acidosis, shock.
CXR	May be normal; atelectasis, pulmonary edema (alveolar & interstitial infiltrates)
Tx	CPR if needed (see 2015 AHA CPR Guidelines for drowning), O_2 therapy ASAP (maintain SpO_2 > 94%), treat bronchospasm, treat hypothermia if present, treat respiratory failure with O_2, NPPV, MV with PEEP, (treat ARDS). Use PEEP early (especially if O_2 > 40%). Treat cerebral edema with diuretics and hyperventilation. Treat pulmonary edema ("secondary drowning") with diuretics and PEEP/CPAP. Watch for arrhythmias, inotropic drugs to improve tissue and cerebral perfusion? Antibiotics? (If infected source).

ORNITHOSIS (PSITTACOSIS, PARROT FEVER)

Def	Atypical pneumonia transmitted to humans from birds
	Inhalation of gram-negative bacterium *Chlamydia psittaci*, which inhabits excrement of Psitticine birds (parrots, cockatoos, lorikeets) infected with *C. psittaci*.
CM	Asymptomatic to severe pneumonia. Cough with scanty, mucoid sputum progressing to mucopurulent, hemoptysis, dyspnea, tachypnea, hypoxemia (severe), chest pain, constitutional symptoms, respiratory failure
CXR	Variable, but may reveal patchy or lobar consolidation
Tx	Antibiotics (tertracycline, erythromycin) and bronchial hygiene

OXYGEN TOXICITY

Def	Pulmonary and systemic damage and injury caused by prolonged inhalation of an elevated P_IO_2.
	Pulmonary oxygen toxicity (normobaric conditions): O_2 less than 40% may never show effects, 100% may show effects within 24 hrs. **CNS (systemic) oxygen toxicity** (hyperbaric conditions)
CM	**Pulmonary** - first-sign: symptoms of acute tracheobronchitis, substernal discomfort, dry hacking cough, vomiting, nausea, tachypnea, hypopnea, chest pain, then progressing to ARDS and pulmonary fibrosis. **CNS** - convulsions, nausea, dizziness, vision/hearing abnormalities, muscle twitching, anxiety, confusion, hiccups, fatigue.
CC	See Oakes' Neonatal/Pediatric Respiratory Care for special considerations related to oxygenation in Neonates
Tx	Keep F_IO_2 less than 0.4 if possible.

PECTUS CARINATUM (PIGEON CHEST)

Def	Outward bending of the anterior ribs forcing sternum outward and increasing AP diameter (convex appearance)
Etiology	Congenital, rickets, kyphoscoliosis, A or V septal defect.
CM	Usually asymptomatic; when symptomatic: decreased stamina/ endurance, frequent respiratory infections, chest pain.
Tx	Usually none; cosmetic or corrective surgery

PECTUS EXCAVATUM (FUNNEL CHEST)

Def	Posterior displacement of the lower sternum (concave appearance)
Etiology	Congenital
CM	Usually asymptomatic, unless severe, then ↓ stamina/endurance, cardiac palpitations during exercise; restrictive lung disease
CXR	Broadened cardiac silhouette
Tx	Usually none; cosmetic or corrective surgery

PLEURAL EFFUSION (HYDROTHORAX)

Def	Excessive accumulation of pleural fluid

Types	**Chylothorax**: chyle **Hemothorax**: blood **Hydrothorax**: serous fluid **Pyothorax**: pus

Etiology	**Transudation**: Plasma passing from vessels into pleural space due to hydraulic or osmotic abnormalities (↓ proteins, ↓ LDH). Causes: atelectasis, CHF, hypoproteinemia, lymphatic obstruction, liver cirrhosis, nephrotic syndrome, pericarditis. **Exudation**: Inflammatory effusion resulting from capillary damage or lymphatic blockage (↑ proteins, ↑ LDH). Causes: acute pancreatitis, cancer, drugs, infections (TB), post-MI syndrome, pulmonary embolism, rheumatoid arthritis, sarcoidosis, SLE. **Note**: See empyema

CM	Dependent on amount of fluid: dyspnea, cough, pain, ↑RR, orthopnea, ↓ BS, egophony, ↓ fremitus, dull to percussion (on affected side), progressing to tracheal deviation and CV compromise with massive effusion > 300 mL.

CXR	Radiopacity of involved cavity and blunting of costophrenic angle, mediastinal shift.

Tx	Depends on size of effusion and symptomology: • If small and/or minimal symptoms, may just be observed • Oxygen Therapy, as needed • Treat underlying cause (see causes above in Etiology) • Thoracentesis or Thoracostomy Tube • Pleurodesis* (malignancy) • Shunt

*Pleurodesis is the process by which a chemical or medication is inserted between 2 layers of pleura, causing them to adhere to each other, with the goal of preventing recurring pleural effusions.

PLEURITIS (PLEURISY)

Def	Inflammation of the pleura
Etiology	Bacterial or viral pneumonia, pleural effusion, pneumothorax, pulmonary emboli, SLE, neoplasms, pulmonary abscess, TB
CM	Abrupt onset; sharp, stabbing pain aggravated by insp. or cough, often unilateral + localized, SOB, intercostal tenderness, splinting, pleural friction rub, infection evid. (if cause).
CXR	Thickening of pleura
Tx	Correct underlying cause

PNEUMOCONIOSIS

Def	Lung disease caused by inhalation of inorganic dust &/ or chemical fumes (See also Hypersensitivity pneumonia: organic).
Etiology	Type of inorganic dust Nonreactive dust: coal (coal-workers lung, black lung) tin, iron (siderosis), barium (baritosis), cement, antimony, titanium Fibrogenic dust (nodular): silica (silicosis), aluminum or magnesium silicate Diffuse: asbestos fibers (asbestosis), aluminum oxide, beryllium, hard metals
CM	Asymptomatic to death – Dependent on type and concentration of dust/fumes, host susceptibility, length of exposure, deposition factors, particle size.
CC	**See Oakes' Ventilator Management (Restrictive Disorders) for Mechanical Ventilation Strategies**
Tx	Avoid causative agent. Also, treat symptoms, O_2 therapy, bronchodilators, steroids

PNEUMOCYSTIS PNEUMONIA (PCP, PNEUMOCYSTOSIS)

Def	Pneumonia caused by the organism *P. jirovecii*, primarily occurring in immunocompromised patients. See AIDS.
	Pneumocystis jirovecii (a fungus); contagious and acquired by patients with depressed cellular immunity or antibody formation from asymptomatic carriers. (Previously called P. carinii)
CM	Slow progression to severe dyspnea and tachypnea, cyanosis, anxiety, concurrent bacterial infection is common, dry cough, fever, PFTs – restrictive.
CXR	Massive consolidation spreading from hilar through most of lung.
EBG	Guidelines for the Prevention and Treatment of Opportunistic Infections in HIV-Infected Adults and Adolescents
Tx	Trimethoprim-sulfamethoxazole (TMP-SMZ), atovaquone, pentamidine, antiretroviral therapy, corticosteroids, O_2 therapy, MV.

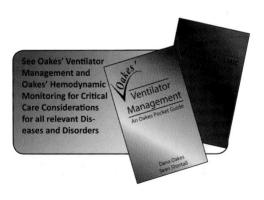

See Oakes' Ventilator Management and Oakes' Hemodynamic Monitoring for Critical Care Considerations for all relevant Diseases and Disorders

Oakes'
Ventilator Management
An Oakes Pocket Guide

Dana Oakes
Sean Shortall

PNEUMONIAS (PNA)

Def	Inflammatory process of the lung's air spaces. Diagnosed by CXR infiltrate, plus 2 or more of: fever, ↑ WBC, &/or purulent sputum.

Types	**Lobar** - air-space inflammation often affecting entire lobe **Broncho** - inflammation of alveoli and contiguous bronchi **Interstitial** - Pneumonitis

Causes:

• Aspiration • Bacterial (TB) • Fungal • Hypersensitivity • Viral	See each type for specifics and treatments

Sources:

Healthcare-Associated	HCAP	• Any Pt hospitalized 2+ days within 90 days of infection • Received recent IV Antibiotics, Chemotherapy, or wound care within past 30 days of infection • Attended hospital or hemodialysis Clinic
Hospital Acquired	HAP	• PNA that occurs > 48 hrs after admission (not incubating at admission)
Ventilator Associated	VAP	• PNA that occurs > 48-72 hrs after endotracheal intubation
Community Acquired	CAP	• Those not meeting any of the above definitions

EBG	Management of Adults with Hospital-Acquired and Ventilator-Associated Pneumonia: 2016 Clinical Practice Guidelines by the Infectious Diseases Society of America and the American Thoracic Society

PNEUMOTHORAX (& AIR LEAK SYNDROME)

Def	Accumulation of gas in the pleural space or other thoracic areas, usually with associated lung collapse	

Types	Spontaneous	no obvious causative event - spont. rupture of bleb/bullae on viseral pleura
	1°	no identifiable lung disease
	2°	pre-existing lung disease
	Traumatic	Includes Iatrogenic and Other
	Indirect	Barotrauma (excessive pressure), often as a result of mechanical ventilation (esp in presence of reduced compliance)
	Direct	Related to Rib fx, surgery, thoracentesis, Line insertions, tracheostomy, etc.
	Tension	Pneumothorax of any cause where air leaks into the pleural cavity, but can't escape - "one-way valve" resulting in a pressure > atmospheric during breathing cycle – **acute medical emergency.**
	Pneumo-Pericardium	Accumulation of gas in the pericardial sac
	Pneumo-Mediastinum	Accumulation of gas in the mediastinum

- BP fistula
- Cancer
- COPD
- Necrotizing pneumonia
- Tuberculosis
- Spontaneous or traumatic (See below).

CM	Asymptomatic to sudden onset of dyspnea, anxiety, ↑RR, ↑ HR, cyanosis, hypoxemia, pleuritic pain (sharp), subcut. emphysema, ↑A-a gradient **Both tension & non-tension:** ↓BS, ↓fremitus, hyperresonance, enlarged hemithorax with ↓ chest expansion (all same side). **Tension:** tympany (same side), mediastinal/tracheal shift (opposite side), severe CV compromise, JVD. **Clinically stable:** RR < 24/min, HR 60-120/min, BP normal, SaO₂ > 90%, patient can speak in whole sentences between breaths. (unstable = lacking these characteristics)
CXR	Air in pleural space or mediastinum, ↑ radiolucency, lung collapse (towards hilar on affected side), absent bronchovascular markings Tracheal/mediastinal shift away from affected side and flattened diaphragm, if tension. **Small spontaneous** = < 3 cm apex-to-cupola **Large spontaneous** = > 3 cm apex-to-cupola
EBG	**Management of Spontaneous Pneumothorax, American College of Chest Physicians Delphi Consensus Statement**
CC	• See **Oakes' Ventilator Management** for in-depth information on pneumothoraces, particularly Barotrauma • See **Oakes' Neonatal/Pediatric Respiratory Care** for in-depth information on Air Leak Syndromes including barotrauma

Tx	Tension pneumothorax requires an EMERGENT THORACENTESIS
	
	Spontaneous pneumothorax:
	Clinically stable with small pneumothorax:
	  1°: observe
	  2°: observe and/or aspirate or chest tube
	Clinically stable with large pneumothorax:
	  2°: re-expand lung with catheter or chest tube
	Clinically unstable with any size pneumothorax:
	  2°: re-expand lung with catheter or chest tube
	Recurrent pneumothorax:
	  Thoracoscopy, pleurodesis, or bullectomy

	PULMONARY EDEMA (CARDIAC ASTHMA)
Def	Accumulation of vascular fluid in alveoli or pulmonary interstitium
Types	Interstitial – Fluid moves only into the interstitium Alveolar – Fluid moves into the interstitium, plus the alveoli.
Etiology	 *Transudation*: due to a vol- ume/ pressure overload of the pulmonary circulation *Causes*: acute MI, ar- rhythmias, CHF, infection, hypervolemia, LVF, renal failure, shock, valve disease	*Exudation*: due to an ↑perme- ability of the pulmonary capillary membrane. *Causes*: ARDS, CNS (hemor- rhage, trauma, stroke, tu- mors, ↑ ICP), near drowning, smoke inhalation, O₂ toxicity
CM	Varies with severity of underlying disorder (↑severity as ↑ fluid). **General**: Sudden anxiety, restlessness, orthopnea, cyanosis, hypoxemia, diaphoresis **Resp**: ↑ RR, dyspnea, cough (dry to pink, frothy fluid), basal crackles/wheezing, SOB, PND, ↓ C **CV**: ↑ HR, ↓ BP, cold clammy skin, JVD, peripheral edema (See also page 1-17 and 8-12)
CXR	**Interstitial**: Haziness of vasculature and hilar **Alveolar**: Irregular, poorly defined ascinar shadows forming a "butterfly" or "bat wing" pattern. **Both**: Disparity between upper and lower lobe venous calibers. LVH when due to CHF. Air-bronchograms
CC	• See **Oakes' Ventilator Management** for Mechanical Venti- lation Strategies • See **Oakes' Hemodynamic Monitoring** for further informa- tion on cardiopulmonary function
Tx	Treat underlying cause. O₂ as needed, diuretics, inotropes and afterload reducing agents, morphine, CPAP, BIPAP, MV with PEEP, cardioversion/resuscitation if needed.

PULMONARY EMBOLISM (PULMONARY INFARCTION)

Def

Blockage of part of pulmonary vascular bed by blood-borne material, sometimes causing pulmonary infarction (necrosis).

Blood (clots, thrombi)(90%):
 Blood stasis – bedrest, CHF, obesity, pregnancy, birth-control pills, post-op
 Vessel wall abnorm.: trauma, phlebitis, infection/parasites
 Abnormal blood coagulation – ↑ clotting or ↓ lysis of clots
Air - CVP line placement
Fat (bone marrow) -fractures, esp. leg bones
Foreign material - drug abuse, indwelling catheters, tumors

CM

EBM suggests using a validated prediction scoring system before proceeding with testing for PE. Wells Scoring System and Revised Geneva Scoring System are common.

Revised Geneva Scoring System, Summarized

Risk Factors	Age > 65 y	1
	Previous DVT or PE	3
	General Anes. or Fx of ↓ Extrem in last month	2
	Acute malignant condition	2
Sympt.	Unilateral lower limb pain	3
	Hemoptysis	2
Clinical	HR 75-94	3
	HR > 95	5
	Pain on lower limb and Unilateral edema	4

Low (0-3), Intermediate (4-10), High (11+)

General	Sudden anxiety, orthopnea, restlessness, cyanosis, possibly leg swelling and pain
Respiratory	dyspnea & sharp chest pain (two most common), ↑ RR, cough (nonproductive to hemoptysis), crackles, wheeze, friction rub,↓ BS, splinting, PFTs – restrictive
CV	↑HR, hypoxemia leading to cor pulmonale

11-59

CXR	Often normal. May have ↑ pulmonary artery size, abrupt tapering of occluded artery, consolidation (atelectasis or infarction), line shadows.
EBG	Antithrombotic Therapy and Prevention of Thrombosis: ACCP Evidence-Based Clinical Practice Guidelines Venous Thromboembolism Diagnosis and Treatment - ICSI Health Care Guideline
	See **Oakes' Hemodynamic Monitoring** for detailed cardiopulmonary function aspects
Tx	• Prophylaxis • O₂ therapy • Treat anxiety/pain • Anticoagulant therapy (heparin & warfarin) • Fibrinolytic therapy (alteplase & reteplase) • Blood Type: Thrombolytic therapy (urokinase & streptokinase) • Fat Type: Steroids • Embolectomy?

RESPIRATORY FAILURE
(ACUTE RESPIRATORY FAILURE, ARF)

Def	Inability of the respiratory system to maintain normal O_2 uptake and CO_2 removal, i.e., failure to maintain gas exchange.
	Hypoxemic: Type I, lung failure, oxygenation failure, or respiratory insufficiency. **Hypercapnic**: Type II, pump failure, or ventilatory failure.
	Any disease or disorder which compromises the ability of the lungs to provide sufficient O_2/CO_2 exchange.

	Hypoxemic	Hypercapnic
CM	$PaO_2 < 60$ mm Hg on FiO_2 $\geq .50$ or $PaO_2 < 40$ mm Hg (any FiO_2) $SaO_2 < 90\%$; Plus, signs and symptoms of hypoxemia (see O_2 Therapy, Chapter 10)	Acute ↑ in $PaCO_2 > 50$ mm Hg with concurrent ↓ in pH < 7.30 (or $PaCO_2$ acutely above baseline in CO_2 retainers) Plus, signs and symptoms of hypercapnia (see Oakes' ABG Pocket Guide)

	Complete critical care coverage of Respiratory Failure can be found in Oakes' Ventilator Management
Tx	Both: Treat underlying cause , O_2 therapy, NPPV or MV, fluid and nutritional management

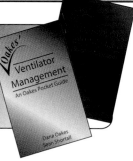

See Oakes' Ventilator Management and Oakes' Hemodynamic Monitoring for Critical Care Considerations for all relevant Diseases and Disorders

Oakes'
Ventilator Management
An Oakes Pocket Guide

Dana Oakes
Sean Shortall

	RESTRICTIVE LUNG DISEASE (DISORDER)
Def	Disease/disorder characterized by a ↓lung volumes/capacities

	Parenchymal conditions:
	  Compression - fibrosis, pleural effusion, pneumothorax, tumor
	  Infiltration - edema, infection, secretions, hyaline membranes
	  Loss of volume - atelectasis, ARDS, ↓surfactant, lobectomy
	  Replacement -fibrous tissue, tumors, etc
	Chest wall abnorm. – musculoskeletal/neuromusc. disorders
	Nervous system control – depression of drive, paralysis

CM	Dyspnea, hypoxemia leading to cor pulmonale, polycythemia, cyanosis, respiratory alkalosis/acidosis (late). ↓ lung volumes (VC ↓ more then FRC and RV), ↓C, normal flows (FEV₁, FVC)
Tx	Treat underlying disease

	SARCOIDOSIS
Def	Relatively benign multisystem, chronic non-caseating granulomatous disorder of undetermined etiology.
	Unknown
CM	Asymptomatic to death. Primarily affects the lungs. Dyspnea, severe cough, scanty mucoid sputum, hypoxemia leading to cor pulmonale, respiratory alkalosis, crackles, constitutional symptoms, spontaneous pneumothorax, PFTs –restrictive.
CXR	Varies greatly
Tx	Tx symptoms, steroids to reduce inflammation; avoid calcium-rich food, vitamin D, sunlight, dusts, chemicals, and fumes

SEVERE ACUTE RESPIRATORY SYNDROME (SARS)	
Def	A contagious, severe respiratory illness (pneumonia) caused by a coronavirus, called SARS-associated coronavirus (SARS-CoV).
CM	Asymptomatic to death. Initial symptoms are flu-like; fever >100.4°F (>38°C), myalgia, sore throat, clinical findings of respiratory illness (dry cough, SOB, difficulty breathing, +/or hypoxia), and potentially evidence of pneumonia, or respiratory distress syndrome
CXR	Patchy, interstitial infiltrates, possible consolidation.
Tx	Respiratory isolation, no specific treatment recommendations at this time; treat symptoms, acquired pneumonia, and any respiratory failure.

DISEASES

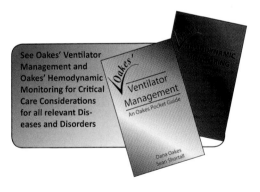

See Oakes' Ventilator Management and Oakes' Hemodynamic Monitoring for Critical Care Considerations for all relevant Diseases and Disorders

Oakes' Ventilator Management
An Oakes Pocket Guide

Dana Oakes
Sean Shortall

SHOCK	
Def	Inadequate tissue perfusion resulting in hypoxic insult and causing widespread abnormal cell metabolism and membrane dysfunction.
	Anaphylactic – Systemic allergic rx causing circulatory failure **Cardiogenic** – Systemic hypoperfusion due to heart failure **Hypovolemic** – ↓ effective circulating volume (most common) **Neurogenic** – Sympathetic NS dysfunction resulting in massive peripheral vasodilation or hypoperfusion **Septic** (vasogenic) – Relative hypovolemia caused by any infection.

Anesthetics, blood, drugs, foods, pollens, venoms	Acute MI, severe hypoxemia, arrhythmias, post-op failure, tension pneumothorax, valve dysfunction	Burns, dehydration, hemorrhage, sepsis, trauma

Anesthesia, brain trauma, drugs, insulin shock, severe pain

Acute pancreatitis, major trauma (including burns) hospital-acquired gram-negative bacilli or gram-positive cocci, fungal infection, immunoincompetence

CM	Varies according to etiology. Diaphoresis, cool clammy, moist skin, agitation, confusion, skin appears gray, dusky, or cyanotic, peripheral pulse rapid & weak, prolonged capillary refilling time, rapid shallow breathing, low to no urine output, chest pain, dizziness, unconsciousness
	See **Oakes' Hemodynamic Monitoring** for detailed cardiopulmonary function aspects of each type of shock
Tx	Correct primary problem, O_2 and ventilation as needed, optimize CO and tissue perfusion.

SLEEP APNEAS

Def	Frequent cessation of breathing during sleep for ≥10 sec.

	Obstructive (OSA)	Central (CSA)
	Anatomic obstruction of upper airway. Ventilatory efforts continue.	Cessation of inspiratory efforts.
	Mixed – Combination of OSA and CSA.	
	Obesity, micrognathia, macroglossia, tonsillar hypertrophy, small or unstable pharynx	Exact etiology unknown; contributing conditions: CHF, stroke, brain lesions, cerebrovascular diseases
CM	Snoring and apnea with increasingly desperate efforts to inhale. May awaken gasping for air. PFTs-obstructive	Mild snoring and apnea
	BOTH: Daytime somnolence, memory loss, personality changes, depression, inability to concentrate, decreased mental acuity, potential arrhythmias, pulmonary hypertension.	
CXR	May develop RHF or LHF	
	Polysomnography (sleep study), avoid sleeping supine, avoid alcohol, sedatives, and REM inhibitors. O_2 therapy as needed.	
Tx	CPAP, BIPAP, tongue retainer, weight reduction, surgery	Pressure ventilation (time cycled) Negative pressure ventilation? Phrenic nerve pacemaker?

SMOKE INHALATION (PULMONARY BURNS)

Def
Inhalation of smoke, fumes, or caustic agents into the tracheo-bronchial tree with potential tissue injury due to heat or toxins.

CM

Signs and Symptoms of Respiratory Tract Injury
Facial burns, singed nasal hairs, reddened pharynx, hoarseness, cough, soot deposits, sooty sputum, central cyanosis, crackles, wheezes, stridor.   Bronchoscopy is gold std for diagnosis.
SpO2 can be profoundly inaccurate in the presence of increased HbCO levels - smoke inhalation. (See CO poisoning)

Stages
Stage I – Acute respiratory distress (wheezing/stridor, ↑RR, hoarseness, cough), may occur in a few hrs, resembles upper airway obstruction
Stage II – Pulmonary edema (8-36 hrs)
Stage III – Bacterial pneumonia (2 days – 3 weeks after injury)

CXR
Variable:
  Normal (Stage I),
  Pulmonary edema/ARDS (Stage II),
  Infiltrates (Stage 3)

CC
* See **Oakes' Ventilator Management** for Mechanical Ventilation Strategies

Tx
Begin 100% O2 to all patients (hyperbaric if CO poison), ensure adequate airway, laryngoscopy or bronchoscopy, closely monitor VS and I&O, , vigorous bronchial hygiene, bronchodilators - racemic epi?, pain meds?, corticosteroids?, Interpercussive Ventilation (IPV)

Burns to face, neck, oropharynx are all indicators to consider early intubation (airway swelling may not appear immediately following insult, but is likely to progress quickly once process begins)

Treat complications: ARDS, burns, pul edema, pneumonia, respiratory failure, shock

TRACHEAL-ESOPHAGEAL FISTULA (T-E FISTULA)

Def	Abnormal passage between trachea and esophagus
	Often congenital, can be iatrogenic ~85% may also have Esophageal Atresia (EA)

CM	Three C's — Choking, Coughing, Cyanosis
	    Excess salivation, aspiration
	    Gastric distention

Tx	• NPO — Provide parenteral nutrition • Position Patient for patent airway and optimum ventilation • Aspirate secretions from oropharynx and pouch • Prevent aspiration • Surgical correction • CPAP is contraindicated (causes severe gastric distension)

See **BP Fistula** in Oakes' Ventilator Management

TRACHEO-INNOMINATE FISTULA (T-I FISTULA)

Def	Abnormal passage between trachea and innominate artery
	Most likely complication from tracheostomy
CM	Bleeding from trach (should inspect quickly) Signs/Symptoms of Shock (see Shock)
Tx	• **This is a Life-Threatening Medical Emergency** • Inspect via Bronchoscopy - URGENT • Either overinflate cuff or digitally compress (with finger) • Surgical Intervention (rapid) • Very often is fatal

TUBERCULOSIS (TB)

Def	Chronic necrotizing bacterial infection, characterized by the formation of tubercles in the lung.
	Miliary TB - hematogenous disssem. throughout the body.
	Mycobacterium tuberculosis. inhalation of droplet nuclei. *Predisposing factors*: malnutrition, diabetes, immunosuppression, HIV, CA, drug/etoh abuse, general debil., steroids
CM	Asymptomatic (majority) to death. Cough with mucoid or mucopurulent sputum, hemoptysis, chest tightness with dull pain, dyspnea, fatigue, fever, irritability, crackles/wheezes/bronchial BS, constitutional symptoms.
CXR	Variable with stage and type, often apical infiltrates with cavities.
EBG	**Evidence-Based Guidelines for the Evaluation, Treatment and Management of TB from WHO, ATS, CDC, and IDSA**
Tx	Use AIRBORNE Precautions, including a Negative-Pressure containment area. Anti-tuberculin drugs (Isoniazid, rifampin, pyrazinamide, ethambutol, streptomycin)

VIRAL PNEUMONIA

Def	Pneumonia caused by viruses
	Most all types. Esp. influenza, adeno, respiratory syncytial, and parainfluenza. *Mycoplasma pneumoniae*: viral like organism (use respiratory isolation), most common cause of nonbacterial pneumonia.
CM	Prior ↑ Resp Infection, dry cough, fever, DOE, cyanosis, fatigue, sore throat
CXR	Variable
Tx	Treat symptoms, if severe, treat like ARDS; bed rest, hydration

12 Pharmacology

PHARM

Always check *manufacturers' inserts for changes in drug information to include dosages, indications, warnings, precautions and contraindications.*

This table is not all-inclusive, and dosages listed are adult dosages, unless indicated. Adult dose is often suitable for children > 12 years of age or > 40kg.

...Oakes' Ventilator Management for detailed information on Critical Care Drugs, including Diuretics, Anticoagulants, Paralytics and Paralytic-Reversal Drugs

Oakes'
✓ Ventilator
Management
An Oakes Pocket Guide

Dana Oakes
Sean Shortall

RESPIRATORY MEDICATION INDEX (PAGE FOUND IN CHAPTER)

Anti-Asthma	
Mast-Cell Stabilizers (14)	• **cromolyn Na**
Anti-Leukotrienes (15)	• **montelukast** (Singular) • **zafirlukast** (Accolate) • **zileuton** (Zyflo)

Bronchodilators	
SABA (16)	• **albuterol** (Accuneb, ProAir-Proventil, Ventolin, Vospire) • **levalbuterol** (Xopenex) • **pirbuterol acetate** (Maxair)
LABA (18)	• **arformoteral tartrate** (Brovana) • **formoterol fumarate** (Foradil, Perforomist) • **salmeterol** (Serevent) • **indacaterol maleate** (Arcapta) • **olodaterol** (Striverdi Respimat)
Anticholinergics (20)	• **aclidinium bromide** • **ipratropium bromide** (Atrovent) • **tiotropium bromide** (Spiriva) • **umeclidinium** (Incruse Ellipta)
Xanthines (21)	• **aminophylline**

Alpha-1 Antitrypsin (22) (proteinase inhibitor)

Anti-Infectives (23)
• **aztreonam** (Cayston) • **colistimethate Na** (Coly-Mycin) • **pentamidine isethionate** (Nebupent) • **ribavirin** (Virazole) • **tobramycin** (Tobi) • **zanamivir** (Relenza)

CF TransMembrane Conductance Regulator Potentiator (26)
• **ivacaftor** (Kalydeco)

IgE Blockers (27)
• **omalizumab** (Xolair) • **reslizumab** (Cinqair) • **mepolizumab** (Nucala)

PHARM

Mucoactives (27)

- **acetylcysteine** (Mucomyst, Mucosol)
- **dornase alfa-DNase** (Pulmozyme)

Inhaled Analgesics (28)

- **lidocaine**
- **morphine sulfate**

Inhaled Epinephrine (29)

- **racemic epinephrine** (S2)

Phosphodiesterase Inhibitors (30)

- **roflumilast** (Daliresp)

Pulmonary Vasodilator (30)

- **Iloprost** (Ventavis) and others

Smoking Cessation (31) drugs

Steroids (34)

- **beclomethasone** (QVAR)
- **budesonide** (Pulmicort Turbuhaler, Pulmicort Respules)
- **ciclesonide** (Alvesco)
- **fluticasone** (Flovent, Arnuity Ellipta)
- **mometasone furoate** (Asmanex)

Wetting Agents (34) (water, salines)

Corticosteroid & LABA (35)

- **budesonide & formoterol** (Symbicort)
- **fluticasone and salmeterol** (Advair)
- **mometazone and formoterol** (Dulera)

Anticholinergic and SABA (36)

- **ipratropium bromide & albuterol** (Combivent, Duoneb)

Anticholinergic and LABA (37)

- **umeclidinium and vilanterol** (Anoro Ellipta)
- **glycopyrrolate and formoterol** (Bevespi Aerosphere)
- **tiotropium and olodaterol** (Stiolto Respimat)
- **glycopyrrolate and indacterol** (Utibron Neohaler)

Abbreviations used in Prescriptions

Aa, aa	of each	IM	intra-muscular	Qid	4x/day
ac	before meals	IV	intra-vascular	Q2h	every 2 hours
ad	to, up to	I&O	intake & output	q3h	every 3 hours
ad lib	as much as needed	L	liter/left	q4h	every 4 hours
aq dist	distilled H2O	m	mix	qs, QS	as much as required
bid	2x/day	mixt	mixture	qt	quart
c̄	with	mL	milliliter	Rx	take
caps	capsule	nebul	spray	s	without
dil	dilute	non rep	not to be repeated	sig	write
el, elix	elixir	NPO	nothing by mouth	sol	solution
emuls	emulsion	ol	oil	solv	dissolve
et	and	p̄	after	sos	if needed (1x)
ext	extract	part acq	equal parts	ss	half
fl, fld	fluid	pc	after meals	stat	immediately
Ft, ft	make	po	by mouth	syr	syrup
gel	gel, jelly	prn	as needed	tab	tablet(s)
g, gm	gram	rect	rectally	tid	3x/day
gr	grain	pulv	powder	tinct	tincture
gtt	drop/drip	q	every	ung	ointment
ht	hypodermic tablet	qh	every hour	ut dict	as directed

Note: see next page for the JCAHO DO NOT USE list.

Medication Abbreviation Do-Not-Use List

Due to high likelihood of errors (similar abbreviations), JCAHO (jointcommission.org) has established a "Do Not Use" list. Currently this does not officially apply to electronic medical records.

Excluded Abbreviations	Recommendation
U (unit)	Write "unit"
IU (International Unit)	Write "International Unit"
Q.D., QD, q.d., qd (daily)	Write: daily
Q.O.D., QOD, q.o.d., qod (every other day)	Write: Every Other Day
*A Trailing 0 (X.0 mg) A lack of leading 0 (.X mg)	Write: X mg (no 0 after decimal) Write: 0.X mg (use 0 before decimal)
MS, MSO$_4$, MgSO$_4$	Write "morphine sulfate" or Write "magnesium sulfate"

*Note that certain things are exempt from the use of a trailing zero, including lab results that show precision (pH 7.0), tube/catheter sizes (ET Tube 8.0), and imaging studies.

Percentage Concentration of Solutions (weight to volume)

%	Ratios	g/L	g/100mL	g/mL	mg/100mL	mg/mL
100	1:1	1000	100	1	100,000	1000
10	1:10	100	10	0.1	10,000	100
5	1:20	50	5	0.05	5,000	50
1	1:100	10	1	0.01	1,000	10
0.5	1:200	5	0.5	0.005	500	5
0.1	1:1000	1	0.1	0.001	100	1

Medication Adminisration Procedures

Every time you administer medications, you should be following these procedures, in addition to using a barcode or similar safety system:

1. Review patient medical record, verifying doctor's orders, code status, allergies, etc.
2. Assure you have the **right medication**.
3. Assure you have the **right dose** (including concentration).
4. Assure you have the **right time**.
5. Assure you have the **right route** (MDI vs. DPI vs. Neb).
6. Verify **right patient** (check I.D. bracelet, DOB).
7. Complete an adequate pre-, mid-, and post assessment.
8. Document administration in a timely manner.

Major Red Flag Drugs

(high potential for Drug-Drug interactions)

• Aspirin	• Theophylline
• Cimetidine	• Warfarin
• Penytoin	

Solving Dosage of Liquids, Tablets, and Capsules

1. Convert all measurements to the same unit

2. $\dfrac{\text{Original Strength}}{\text{Amount Supplied}} = \dfrac{\text{Desired Strength (dosage)}}{\text{Unknown amount to be supplied}}$

Example 1:	Example 2:
How many mL of a drug must be given to deliver 75,000 units (50,000 units/mL)?	How many mLs of a drug, at a concent. of 25 mg/mL of solution, would be needed to provide 100 mg?
$\dfrac{50,000}{\text{mL}} = \dfrac{75,000}{\text{X mL}}$	$\dfrac{25 \text{ mg}}{\text{mL}} = \dfrac{100 \text{ mg}}{\text{X mL}}$
$X = \dfrac{75,000}{50,000} = 1.5 \text{ mL}$	$X = \dfrac{100 \text{mg}}{25 \text{ mg}} = 4 \text{ mL}$

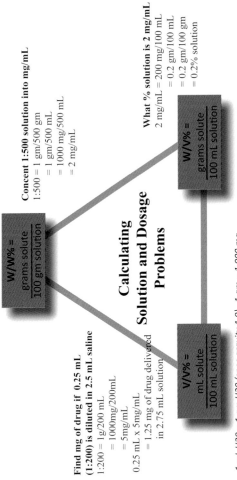

Calculating Solution and Dosage Problems

Concent 1:500 solution into mg/mL

1:500 = 1 gm/500 gm
= 1 gm/500 mL
= 1000 mg/500 mL
= 2 mg/mL

What % solution is 2 mg/mL

2 mg/mL = 200 mg/100 mL
= 0.2 gm/100 mL
= 0.2 gm/100 gm
= 0.2% solution

$$W/W\% = \frac{grams\ solute}{100\ gm\ solution}$$

$$W/V\% = \frac{grams\ solute}{100\ mL\ solution}$$

$$V/V\% = \frac{mL\ solute}{100\ mL\ solution}$$

Find mg of drug if 0.25 mL (1:200) is diluted in 2.5 mL saline

1:200 = 1g/200 mL
= 1000mg/200mL
= 5mg/mL
0.25 mL x 5mg/mL
= 1.25 mg of drug delivered in 2.75 mL solution

1 mL H20 = 1 gm H20 (spec gravity 1.0)   1 gm = 1,000 mg

PHARM

12-7

Conversion within Same System

Set up a proportion:	How many mg are in 5 g?
$\dfrac{gm}{mg} = \dfrac{gm}{mg}$	$\dfrac{1\ gm}{1000\ mg} = \dfrac{5\ gm}{X}$

Conversion between Systems

Set up a proportion:	How many grains in 5 g?
$\dfrac{one\ system}{other\ system} = \dfrac{one\ system}{other\ system}$	$\dfrac{metric}{apothecary} = \dfrac{metric}{apothecary}$
	$\dfrac{1\ gm}{15\ grains} = \dfrac{5\ gm}{X}$

Approximate Dosage Equivalents

Metric		Avoirdupois	
1mg	0.015 grain	1 lb	454 gm
1 gm	15 grains	1 ounce	28.4 gm
1 kg	2.2 lbs		
1 mL	16 drops (gtts)		

Apothecary		Household	
1 grain	60 mg	1 teaspoon	5 mL
1 ounce	30 gm	1 tablespoon	15 mL 3 teaspoons
1 fl ounce	30 mL	1 cup	240 mL 8 fl ounces
1 pint	500 mL		
1 quart	1000 mL		
1 gallon	4000 mL		

Adjusting for Pediatric Dosages

Remember that recommended dosages are only estimates. Dosages should be individualized - adjust for variations in maturity, metabolism, temperature, obesity, edema, illness and individual tolerances.

Current literature supports BSA as the most consistent and accurate method of drug dosing over a wide range of body sizes. However, for small children (< 10 kg) dosing should be made on a mg/kg basis as BSA increases disproportionately as weight decreases.

Most drugs are dosed on a mg/kg basis in children. Due to differences in distribution, metabolism, and elimination, children require higher mg/kg dose than adults. While this works well for younger children, in older larger children and adolescents (>40 kg), when dosed by this method, adult doses can often be exceeded.

For this reason:
**never give a child a dose greater
than the usual adult dose,
regardless of height or weight.**

Body Surface Area (Clark's BSA) Rule

Estimated child's dose = $\dfrac{\text{Child's BSA (m}^2\text{) x Adult dose}}{1.73}$

$$\text{BSA (m2)} = \sqrt{\dfrac{\text{height(cm) x weight(kg)}}{3600}}$$

Lamb, TK, Leung, D. More on Simplified Calculation of Body Surface Area. New England Journal of Medicine 1988: 318:1130

Estimation of BSA for Children of "Normal Height and Weight"

Weight		Approximate Age	Surface Area (sq m)
kg	lb		
3	6.6	Newborn	0.2
6	13.2	3 months	0.3
10	22	1 year	0.45
20	44	5.5 years	0.8
30	66	9 years	1
40	88	12 years	1.3
50	110	14 years	1.5
65	143	Adult	1.7
70	154	Adult	1.76

adapted from West's nomogram

Body Weight Rules

Clark's Rule (patients > 2 yrs)

Child's dose = $\dfrac{\text{Body Wt (lbs) x adult dose}}{150}$

Weight-Based Dosing:

Dose = pediatric dose/kg x child's weight (kg)

Age Rules (less accurate than BSA or weight-based)

Fried's Rule (infants up to 24 mos)

Infant's dose = $\dfrac{\text{age (mos) x adult dose}}{150}$

Young's Rule (2-12 yrs)

Child's dose = $\dfrac{\text{age (yrs) x adult dose}}{\text{age (yrs) + 12}}$

PHARM

Bronchodilators

Adrenoreceptor Responses

Receptor	Target
alpha-1	Dilates pupils, contracts smooth muscle
beta-1	Stimulates force/rate of heart
beta-2	Bronchodilator of lungs, causes voluntary muscle tremors

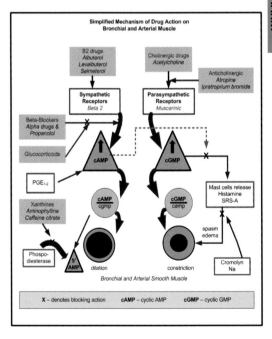

Assessing Response to Bronchodilator Therapy[1]

Indications

Assessment of airflow and other clinical indicators to:
Confirm therapy is approp.
Individualized medication dose &/or frequency
Determine patient status during therapy
Determine need for changes in therapy (dose, frequency, types of medication)

Contraindications

Some assessment maneuvers should be postponed during acute, severe distress.

Hazards/Complications

Airway collapse
Bronchoconstriction
Coughing &/or syncope
Procedures associated

Frequency

Acute, unstable patient –
Pre-therapy: ABGs, full assessment, baseline values
Pre and Post therapy: BS, side effects, vital signs, PEFR, or FEV1 (freq. is based upon acuteness and severity).
Continuous: SpO2

Stable patient-
Hospital: PEF (pre and post therapy initially, then 2 x/ day.
Home: PEF initially 3-4/day than 2x/day, depending on severity of symptoms.

Assessment of Outcome/Monitoring

Pre-therapy (identify):
Clinical indications
Contraindications
Respiratory and CV baseline values

During therapy (identify):
Adverse responses
Clinical changes

Post therapy (identify):
Adverse responses
Therapeutic responses
Lack of therapeutic responses

Trend analysis (identify):
Change in baseline
Need to – change therapy, discontinue therapy, modify dose

Document
Patient responses and progress: breath sounds, lung function (PEFR, FEV, FVC), vital signs, symptoms.

continued next page

Bronchodilator Therapy (continued)

Monitoring	PFT's:
Patient observation: Accessory muscle use decreased General appearance improved Sputum expectoration increased **Auscultation:** BS improved and volume of air moved is increased Vital signs improved Subjective patient improvement	FEV_1 &/or FVC (improved by 12% increase and 200mL increase) &/or FEF 25-75% improved, ↑PEF. SaO_2, SpO_2 &/or ABG's improved Exercise performance improved Ventilator variables improved: Decreased: auto- PEEP, PIP, Pplat, Raw Increased: expiratory flow

1) Adapted from AARC Clinical Practice Guidelines: Assessing Response to Bronchodilator Therapy at Point of Care, *Respiratory Care*, Volume 40, # 12, 1995.

Bronchodilators: Summary of General Side Effects

Pulmonary	Cardiovascular	CNS	Other
Bronchial irritation Bronchial edema	↑BP, ↑HR, anginal pain, coronary insufficiency, palpitations, peripheral vaso- constriction	Anxiety/fear, headache, irritability, insomnia, restlessness, tremor, vertigo, weakness	Hypersensi- tivity, reac- tion to MDI propellants, tachyphylaxis, urinary reten- tion, vomit- ing, nausea

Black Box Warning for LABAs *(see inserts for full warning)*

May increase the risk of asthma-related deaths. Use as a treatment for asthma not controlled with a control drug (such as inhaled corticosteroid). Discontinue LABA as soon as possible after asthma control is attained. Consider use of combination products (e.g. LABA + Corticosteroid).

Anti-Asthma - Mast Cell Stabilizers

Medication	Dosage	Indications/Actions	Contraindications/Notes
cromolyn Na	INHALED SOLUTION: 10 mg/mL – 2 mL vial 2 yr – adult: 20 mg 4x/day may ↓ to 2-3x/day when stable ALLERGEN OR EIA: Administer single dose 10-15 min, but not > 60 min, before precipitating event.	- Prophylactic maintenance of mild to moderate asthma. - Not for acute exacerbations. - Prevention of allergen or EIA *Prevents release of inflammatory mediators from inflammatory cell types.*	Adverse: Bronchospasm, cough, local irritation, dry mouth, chest tightness, vertigo, unpleasant taste in mouth. Neb solution (may dilute) may be mixed with albuterol.

Anti-asthma - Anti-Leukotrienes

Medication	Dosage	Indications/Actions	Contraindications/Notes
montelukast *Singulair*	**Asthma, seasonal or perennial allergic rhinitis (taken in PM):** 12-24 mos: 4 mg granules 1x/day 2-6 yrs: 4 mg 1x/day 6-15 yrs: 5 mg 1x/day Adults: 10 mg: 1x/day **Bronchoconstriction, EIA (prevention):** Granules: 4 mg/packet Chewable Tablet: 4 mg, 5 mg Tablet: 10 mg	**Seasonal/perennial allergic rhinitis, prophylaxis and chronic treatment of asthma, prevention of exercise-induced bronchospasm** *Leukotriene receptor antagonist blocks inflammatory mediators*	**Adverse:** Headache, dizziness, dyspepsia, fatigue. May increase liver function test.
zafirlukast *Accolate*	**5-11 yr:** 10 mg 2x/day **≥ 12 yr:** 20 mg 2x/day Tablet: 10 mg, 20 mg	Prophylaxis/chronic treatment of asthma	Same as above Admin 1 hr before or 2 hr after meals.
zileuton *Zyflo*	**≥ 12 yr:** 600 mg 4x/day (tabs) 1200 mg 2x/day (extended rel)	*Leukotriene inhibitor:* *Prevents formation of inflammatory mediators*	Headache, dizziness, dyspepsia, fatigue, elevated LFT's (≥ 3x upper limit norm)

Bronchodilators: Beta Agonists SABA

Medication	Dosage	Indications/Actions	
albuterol *AccuNeb* *ProAir RespiClick* *Proventil HFA* *Proventil* *Ventolin* *Vospire ER*	See Chart Below	**Bronchoconstriction, Acute and Maintenance** Stimulates β1 (minor), β2 (strong) **Onset:** 5 min. **Peak:** 30-60 min **Duration:** 3-8 hours	**Adverse:** Slight CV and CNS, hyperglycemia, hypokalemia, tremors

ACUTE EXACERBATION (NIH GUIDELINES)

NEBULIZER:
Child: 0.15 mg/kg (minimum 2.5 mg), every 20 min x 3 doses, then
0.15-0.3 mg/kg (up to 10 mg), every 1-4 hrs prn **or**
0.5 mg/kg/hr by continuous neb.
Adult: 2.5-5 mg every 20 min x 3 doses, then 2.5-10 mg,
every 1-4 hrs prn or 10-15 mg/hr by continuous neb.

MDI:
Child: 4-8 puffs, every 20 min x 3 doses, then every 1-4 hrs prn.
Adult: 4-8 puffs, every 20 min (up to 4 hrs), then every 1-4 hrs prn.
MDI (HFA and DPI): 90 mcg/puff
Neb. Soln: 5mg/mL (0.5%); 2.5mg/3mL (0.083%), 1.25mg/3mL
    (0.042%), 0.63mg/3mL (0.021%).
Syrup: 2mg/5mL; Tabs: 2, 4 mg; Extended release tabs: 4, 8 mg

NON-ACUTE (MAINTENANCE)

NEBULIZER:
Child < 12 yrs: 0.15-0.25mg/kg (max 5mg), every 4-6 hrs prn
> 12 yrs: 2.5-5 mg, every 4-6 hrs prn

MDI:
Child < 12 yrs: 1-2 puffs 4x/day
Child > 12 yrs – Adult: 2-4 puffs, every 4-6 hrs
                     (max 12 puffs/day)

ORAL:
2-6 yrs: 0.1-0.2 mg/kg/dose, 3x/day (max 12 mg/day)
6-12 yrs: 2 mg/dose, 3-4x/day,
        extended release 4 mg, 2x/day (max 24 mg/day)
> 12 yrs – Adults: 2-4 mg/dose, 3-4x/day, extended release
                4-8 mg, 2x/day (max 32 mg/day)

Bronchodilators: Beta Agonists SABA

Medication	Dosage	Indications/Actions	
levalbuterol *Xopenex* *Xopenex HFA*	**SOLUTION FOR NEBULIZATION:** 0.31 mg/3mL; 0.63 mg/3 mL; 1.25 mg/0.5 mL; 1.25 mg/3 mL **≤ 4 yrs:** 0.31 -1.25 mg, every 4-6 hr, PRN **5-12 yrs:** 0.31 mg 3x/day (max 0.63 mg 3x/day) **12 + yrs:** 0.63-1.25 mg, 3x/day **MDI: 45 mcg/puff** 4+ yrs: 1-2 puffs, every 4-6 hrs, PRN	**Bronchoconstriction** *R-isomer form of albuterol, stimulates Beta-2 (strong)* **Onset:** 15 min **Peak:** 1.5 hr **Dur:** 5-8 hrs	**Adverse:** Slight CV and CNS effects *(less than with albuterol);* hyperglycemia, hypokalemia Risk of paradoxical bronchospasm
terbutaline *Brethaire* *Brethine* *Bricanyl*	**Not typically used clinically today** **1 mg/mL** < 12 yrs: 0.5 mg/kg 3x/day (max 5 mg/day) 12-15 yrs: 2.5 mg 3x/day (max 7.5 mg/day) > 15 yrs: 5 mg 3x/day; reduce to 2.5 mg 3x/day	**Bronchoconstriction** **Off Label: preterm labor** *Stimulates β-1 (mild), β-2 (mod)*	**Adverse:** Slight CV and CNS, hyperglycemia, hypokalemia, tremors Risk of paradoxical bronchospasm

Bronchodilators: Beta Agonists LABA

Medication	Dosage	Indications/Actions	Contraindications/ Notes
arformoterol tartrate *Brovana*	**Solution for Nebulization:** 15 mcg / 2 mL **Adults:** 15 mcg 2x/day (do not exceed 30 mcg/day)	**Maintenance treatment of COPD** *Selective long-acting β2-adrenergic receptor agonist*	Adverse: slight CV/CNS NOT indicated for acute constriction **Black Box Warning (see pg 12-13)**
formoterol fumarate *Perforomist*	Foradil was discontinued 1/2016 **Solution for Nebulization:** 20 mcg/2 mL **Adults:** 20 mcg every 12 hrs	**Maintenance treatment of COPD** *Long acting selective β2 agonist.* **Onset:** 1-3 min **Peak:** 30-60 min **Duration:** 12 hrs.	Adverse: slight CV/CNS NOT indicated for acute constriction **Black Box Warning (see pg 12-13)**

Bronchodilators: Beta Agonists LABA

Medication	Dosage	Indications/Actions	Contraindications/Notes
salmeterol *Serevent Diskus*	**POWDER:** (50 mcg/dose) > 4 yrs: 1 inh 2x/day, 12 hrs apart for: Asthma (>4 yrs; mainten and prevention) COPD (adults) **PREVENTION OF EIA (> 4yrs):** 1 inh (50 mcg) at least 30 minutes prior to exercise. Don't repeat within 12 hrs, and not to be used by patients on salmeterol 2x/day	**Long-Term management of Bronchoconstriction** *Long acting selective β2 agonist.* **Onset:** 10-20 min **Peak:** 3 hrs. **Duration:** 12 hrs.	**Adverse:** slight CV/CNS NOT indicated for acute constriction **Black Box Warning** (see pg 12-13)
indacaterol *Arcapta Neohaler*	Inhalation capsule: 75 mcg Adults: inhale 75 mcg once daily	**Maintenance treatment of COPD** *Long acting selective β2 agonist.*	NOT indicated for acute constriction
olodaterol *Striverdi Respimat*	2.5 mcg/dose Adults: 2 actuations (= 5 mcg), once daily		**Black Box Warning** (see pg 12-13)

PHARM

12-19

Medication	Dosage	Indications/Actions	
aclidinium bromide *Tudorza Pressair*	400 mcg/inh Adults: 1 inh 2x/day	Maintenance tx of bron-chospasm associated with COPD	Current concerns about administering to patients with underlying cardiovas-cular disease
umeclidinium bromide *Incruse Ellipta*	62.5 mcg per actuation Adults: 1 inh once daily	*Long-acting M3 muscarinic antagonist*	
ipratropium bromide *Atrovent* *Atrovent HFA*	Solution for Nebulization: (0.02%) (0.5 mg/2.5 mL) >12 yr: 0.25-0.5 mg, 3-4x/day <12 hr: 0.25-0.5 mg, 3x/day MDI: (17 mcg/puff) <12 yr: 1-2 puffs, 3x/day (max 6/day) >12 yr: 2-3 puffs, 4x/day (max 12/day)	Treatment of broncho-spasm associated with COPD, bronchitis/emphy-sema *Anticholinergic: blocks acetyl-choline + potentiates β2 stim.* ACUTE EXACERBATION: >12 yrs: 0.5 mg, every 20 min x 3, then every 2-4 hrs <12 yrs: 0.25-0.5 mg, every 20min x 3, then every 2-4 hrs. MDI: (all ages) (NIH Guidelines): 4-8 puffs, every 20 minutes as needed for up to 3 hrs	Adverse: mucus viscosity, local inflammation, dry mouth, pupil dilation **Not to be used as a rescue inhaler**

Xanthines

Medication	Dosage	Indications/Actions	Contraindications/Notes
tiotropium bromide *Spiriva* *(HandiHaler)* *(Respimat)*	**DPI (HANDIHALER):** 18 mcg COPD: 2 inh of 1 cap/day **MDI (RESPIMAT):** 1.25, 2.5 mcg COPD: 2 inh of 2.5 mcg daily Asthma: 2 inh of 1.25 mcg daily	Maintenance tx of COPD Action same as Atrovent **Onset:** 30 min **Peak:** 3 hrs **Duration:** >24 hrs	**Adverse:** dry mouth, urinary retention, constipation, increased HR, blurred vision, glaucoma **Not to be used as a rescue inhaler**

Medication	Dosage	Indications/Actions	Contraindications/Notes
aminophylline	**NEONATAL APNEA:** Load: 5 mg/kg over 30" (IV or PO) Maintenance: 5 mg/kg/day, q 12 hrs **BRONCHODILATION:** Load: 6 mg/kg over 20-30 min (IV) Maintenance: Neonate: 0.2mg/kg/hr; 6 wk - 6 mo: 0.5mg/kg/hr 6mo—12mo: 0.6-0.7 mg/kg/hr	Bronchoconstriction Neonatal apnea Bronchodilation (inhibits phospho- diesterase) *Stimulates rate and depth of resp., pulm. vasodilation* **1-9 yrs:** 1-1.2 mg/kg/hr **9-12 yrs:** 0.9 mg/kg/hr (+ young smokers) **> 12 yrs:** 0.7 mg/kg/hr (+ older nonsmokers)	↑CV and CNS effects, many systemic effects Toxicity > 20 mg/L (>15 mg/L in neonates)

Alpha-1 Antitrypsin Disorder

Medication	Dosage	Indications/Actions	Contraindications/Interactions
Alpha 1 Proteinase Inhibitor *Human*	60 mg/kg once weekly For IV use only, infuse over 30 min. **POWDER FOR RECONSTITUTION:** **Aralast NP:** 500 mg, 1000 mg vials **Prolastin:** 1000 mg vial **Zemaira:** 1000 mg vial **Glassia:** 1000 mg (50 mL) Injection solution	**Congenital alpha 1- antitrypsin deficiency.** *Replaces enzymes lost in patients with this disorder*	Hypersensitivity and anaphylactic reactions **Adverse:** ↑ALT, AST, Headache, Musculoskeletal discomfort, pharyngitis, allergic reactions, fever, light headedness

Anti-Infectives

Medication	Dosage	Indications/Actions	Contraindications/Notes
aztreonam *Cayston*	Powder for Reconstitution: Oral Inhalation (75 mg) ≥ 7 yrs: 75 mg 3x/day x 28 days *Do not repeat for 28 days after completion*	Management of *P. aeruginosa* infection in cystic fibrosis	Administer bronchodilator first Administer alone (do not mix with other nebulized meds) Watch for bronchospasm
colistimethate Na *Coly-Mycin*	Solution for Nebulization: 75mg/mL 50–75 mg every 8-12 hours	**Management of *P. aeruginosa*** *Antibiotic for G-activity (pseudomonal activity)*	Dilute dose in NS to 4 mL Administer via Pari LC plus nebulizer & filter valve set Mix immediately before admin.

Medication	Dosage	Indications/Actions	Considerations
pentamidine isethionate *NebuPent*	- **5+ yrs:** 300 mg (1 vial), q 3-4 wks - **<5 yrs:** 8 mg/kg/dose (up to 300mg) - Deliver via Respirgard II neb at 5-7 LPM at 50 PSI until gone	**Prophylaxis of Pneumocystis pneumonia** *Anti-protozoan*	Do not mix with other drugs Mix 300 mg (1 vial) w/ 6mL sterile water Administer bronchodilator prior to tx **Adverse Reactions:** Irritation, cough, fatigue, SOB, bronchospasm, metallic taste, systemic effects
Note: Caregiver precautions – administer only in an isolated room with separate air circulating system and neg. pressure. Minimize environmental drug exposure. Wear gown, gloves, mask and goggles. Nebulize to <3 µm MMAD.			
ribavirin *Virazole*	**AEROSOL VIA SPAG-2:** 2 grams over 2 hrs 3x/day (60 mg/mL - 6 grams reconstituted w/ 100 mL of sterile, preservatitve-free water, for 3-7 days.	**Severe lower respiratory tract infection** (RSV, Influenza A, B, Herpes) *Antiviral (RSV/Influenza A & B)*	Not recommended for intubated patients Do not mix with other drugs Deliver with SPAG-2
May cause adverse effects in healthcare workers (especially for pregnant women). Use of neg. pressure room, scavenging devices (SPAG), and resp. masks is recommended.		Watch for acute respiratory deterioration + CV effects. Deliver aerosol into mask or hood, (not ET tube and/or vent).	

Medication	Dosage	Indications/Actions	Contraindications/Notes
tobramycin *Tobi*	**AEROSOL:** > 6 yr: 300 mg, every 12 hr (300 mg/5 mL), repeat in cycles: 28 days on, 28 days off <6yr: 100 mg, every 12h	**Management of P. aeruginosa infections in cystic fibrosis patients.** *Antibiotic for G- activity (Pseudomonal activity)*	Don't dilute/mix w/ other drugs. Admin via Pari®LC plus nebulizer + filter valve set Adverse Reactions: multiple (review mfr insert)
zanamivir *Relenza*	POWDER/INHALATION: 5 mg/blister Influenza treatment: ≥ 7 yrs: 10 mg inhaled 2x/day Influenza prophylaxis: ≥ 5 yrs: 10 mg inhaled, 1/day x 10 days	*Treatment of influenza A or B*	Use a dischaler Not recommended for use in patients with airway disease

12-25

Cystic Fibrosis Transmembrane Conductance Regulator (CFTR) Potentiator

Medication	Dosage	Indications/Actions	Contraindications/Notes
Ivacaftor *Kalydeco*	2yrs-6yrs: One 150mg tablet, every 12 hours	*Indicated for the treatment of cystic fibrosis (CF) in patients age 6 years and older who have a G551D mutation in the CFTR gene.* *A cystic fibrosis transmembrane conductance regulator (CFTR) potentiator*	Adverse: URI, headache, stomach ache, rash, diarrhea, and dizziness. It is not effective in CF patients with two copies of the F508 mutation in the CFTR gene, which is the most common mutation that results in CF. If a patient's mutation status is not known, an FDA-cleared CF mutation test should be used to determine whether the G551D mutation is present.

IgE Blockers

Medication	Dosage	Indications/Actions	Contraindications/Notes
omalizumab *Xolair*	Injected drug/weight-based	**Mod-Sev Asthma (adults)** *monoclonal antibody*	Bruising, erythema
reslizumab *Cinqair*	See Prescribing Information for specific dosaging, frequency	**Severe Asthma (adults)** *add-on maintenance tx*	See **Black Box Warning** for this
mepolizumab *Nucala*		**Severe Asthma (adults)** *add-on maintenance tx*	

Mucoactives

Medication	Dosage			Indications/Actions	Contraindications/Notes
acetylcysteine *Mucomyst*	**INHALATION SOLUTION: T-Qid**			**Tenacious mucous** *Breaks mucus disulfide bonds. Decreases mucous viscosity.* Peak: 5-10 min Duration: > 1 hr	**Adverse:** Bronchospasm (administer bronchodilator before use), stomatitis, nausea, rhinitis, unpleasant odor/taste. Overmobilization of secretions
	Age	**10%**	**20%**		
	> 12 yr:	10 mL	5 mL		
	Child:	6-10 mL	3-5 mL		
	Infant:	2-4 mL	1-2 mL		
	20% is diluted 1:1 with H2O or NS				
	INSTILLATION: q 1-4 hrs, prn 1-2 mL (20%) (200 mg/mL) 2-4 mL (10%) (100 mg/mL)				
dornase alfa-dnase *Pulmozyme*	**INHALATION SOLUTION:** 3 mos- adult: 2.5 mg, 1-2 x/day (1 mg/mL, 2.5 mL amp)			**Tenacious mucus (decreases infection)** *Dornase alpha recombinant, decrease viscocity*	Same as acetylcysteine → Do not mix or dilute with other drugs.

12-27

Inhaled Analgesics

Medication	Dosage	Indications/Actions	Contraindications/Notes
Lidocaine (off-label)	Nebulized- 2-4ml of 1%-4% lidocaine. Dosing varies greatly in literature. (Start with lower dosing)	Pre-bronchoscopy. Pre-nasogastric tube insertion. Intractable cough. Has also been used to treat asthma. Inhibits Na ion channels.	Use with caution. May cause airway irritation, reduced gag reflex leading to aspiration.
Morphine Sulfate (off-label)	Nebulized- Starting dose- 2-5mg Q4prn Mix with 3ml normal saline. BAN recommended. (Higher doses and escalating frequency may be needed).	Dyspnea, pain and cough in palliative care patients. Binds to opioid receptors, producing analgesia (opioid agonist).	Use with caution. May cause bronchospasm, respiratory depression, constipation and nausea. May pre-treat with a bronchodilator or have bronchodilator ready. Escalating doses with more frequent treatments may be necessary. Nebulize as an alternate route of delivery other than PO or IV.

Inhaled Epinephrine

Medication	Dosage	Indications/Actions	Contraindications/Notes
Racemic epinephrine *S2* *Asthmanefrin*	INHALATION SOLUTION: 22.5 mg/mL 1 (0.5 mL) dose = 11.25 mg (2.25%) S2: 0.25-0.5 mL (2.25%) diluted in 3 mL NS Stridor (2.25%): < 5 kg: 0.25 mL/dose > 5 kg: 0.5 mL/dose Asthmanefrin: 1-3 inh of 0.5 mL of 2.25% via EZ Breathe atomizer	Bronchoconstriction Tracheobronchial inflammation (post extubation, etc.) Nasal congestion Stimulates: alpha-1 (mild) beta-1 (medium) beta-2 (mild) Duration: ½-2 hrs	Milder effects than epinephrine Rebound airway edema, cardiac arrhythmias, chest pain, trembling, dizziness, headache Use min # doses to get response

PHARM

12-29

Phosphodiesterase Inhibitors

Medication	Dosage	Indications/Actions	Contraindications/Notes
roflumilast *Daliresp*	Adults: 500 mcg PO Once Daily 500 mcg tabs	COPD prophylaxis (reduction in acute exacerbations) Recommended for severe or very severe COPD w/ bronchitic component PDE4 Inhibitor (may affect enzyme that contributes to bronchoconstriction and inflammation)	DO NOT use as a bronchodilator Should not be used for relief of acute bronchospasm Contraindicated in pts with liver impairment, not recommended in tandem with rifampin, carbamezepine, phenytoin, phenobarbital.

Pulmonary Vasodilators

Medication	Dosage	Indications/Actions	Contraindications/Notes
iloprost *Ventavis*	INHALATION SOLUTION: 10 mcg/mL; 20 mcg/mL Initial: 2.5 mcg inhaled, ↑dose to 5 mcg, 6-9 x/day No more than q 2 hr during waking hrs Max/day: 45 mcg	Pulmonary hypertensive arterial disease	Use I-Neb or Prodose AAD System
Other Pulmonary Vasodilators:		epoprostenol (Flolan, Veletri) - IV sildenafil (Revatio) - tab	tadalafil (Adcirca) -tab treprostinil (Tyvaso, Remodulin) – inhal/inject
		ambrisentan (Letairis) - tab bosentan (Tracleer) - tab	

5 A's of Smoking

ASK	every patient should be asked if they use tobacco every time you see them
ADVISE	non-judgmentally, advise all smokers to quit
ASSESS	assess the smoker for motivation (are they ready to quit?)
ASSIST	develop a plan with the smoker to quit, discuss pharmacological options, recommend counseling, provide adequate materials
ARRANGE	directly follow-up on regular intervals, or arrange for adequate follow-up

Fagerstrom Test for Nicotine Dependence

How soon after you wake up do you smoke your first cigarette?	5 min or less 6-30 minutes 31-60 minutes 60+ minutes	3 points 2 points 1 point 0 points
Do you find it hard to refrain from smoking in places where it is forbidden?	Yes No	1 point 0 points
What cigarette would you hate most to give up?	First Morning Any other	1 point 0 point
How many cigarettes per day do you smoke?	10 or less 11-20 21-30 31 or more	0 points 1 point 2 points 3 points
Do you smoke more during the first hours after waking?	Yes No	1 point 0 points
Do you smoke if you are so ill you can't get out of bed?	Yes No	1 point 0 points

≥6 indicates a high level of dependence

Smoking Cessation

Medication	Dosage	Summary of Action	Contraindications/Notes
varenicline *Chantix*	**Start Chantix 1 week prior to quit date.** -1mg 2x/day after a 1 week titration: Days 1-3: 0.5mg daily Days 4-7: 0.5mg 2x/day Day 8+: 1mg 2x/day 12 wk course of treatment, then another 12 weeks if success during 1st course	*Binds with neuronal nicotinic acetylcholine receptors. Produces agonist activity (blocks the reward/reinforcement a person may feel as a result of smoking).*	**Side Effects may be common:** -serious neuropsychiatric symptoms, including changes in behavior, agitation, depressed mood, suicidal ideation and suicidal behavior nausea (mild-moderate, persistent); sleep disturbance, flatulence, constipation.
bupropion *Zyban*	**Tablets** (150 mg) Start 2wks before quitting 150 mg/day x 3 days *then* 150mg 2x/day for 7-12 weeks	*Unknown, may have nonadrenergic or dopaminic effects (decreases some of the cravings for cigarettes)*	Should not be taken with MAO Inhibitors, or people with seizure disorders. **See insert for Black Box Warning**
Nasal Spray *Nicotrol NS*	Nasal Spray (0.5mg nicotine per spray) 1-2 doses per hour, not to exceed 40mg (80 sprays) per day	*Nicotine Replacement therapies decrease with-drawal symptoms by giving measured, smaller doses of nicotine*	Patient should be instructed to not smoke concurrently Use should not exceed 6 mos.

Smoking Cessation

Medication	Dosage	Summary of Action	Contraindications/Notes
Transdermal patch *Nicotrol*	**15 mg/patch for 6 weeks** **>10 cigarettes/day:** Apply 1 patch in the A.M.; remove before bed (don't wear overnight)	*Nicotine Replacement therapies decrease withdrawal symptoms by giving measured, smaller doses of nicotine*	**Adverse:** skin irritation, insomnia **Precautions:** pregnancy, heart disease
Transdermal Patch *Nicoderm CQ*	**Patch 7, 14, 21 mg/patch** <10 cig/day: 14mg for 16-24hr x 6wk *then* 7mg for 16-24hr x 2 wk >10 cig/day: 21mg for 16-24hr x 6wk *then* 14mg for 16-24hr x 2 wk *then* 7mg for 16-24hr x 2 wk		
Gum/ Lozenges *Nicorette Gum, Commit Lozenge*	**Gum:** 2, 4 mg (max: 30 pcs/day) **Lozenges:** 2, 4 mg (max: 20 loz/day) 2-4 mg over 30 min q 1-2 hr x 6wk, *then* q. 2-4 hr x 3 wk, *then* q. 4-8 hr x 3 wk		Dentures Pregnancy Heart Disease
Oral Inhaler *Nicotrol*	10mg cartridges, 4mg delivered 6-16 cartridges per day Patient should be instructed in controlling depth and frequency of inhalation		**Adverse:** dyspepsia, cough, mouth irritation/burning Avoid in COPD, asthma, pregnancy and heart disease

Steroids

Medication	Dosage	Summary of Action	Contraindications/Notes
beclomethasone (QVAR) **budesonide** (Pulmicort, Flexhaler Pulmicort Respules) **fluticasone** (Flovent) (Arnuity Ellipta) **mometasone furoate** (Asmanex) **ciclesonide** (Alvesco)	See insert for dosing information	*Anti-inflammatory* *for maintenance with* *prophylactic treatment* *of asthma*	Cough, sneezing, dysphonia, pharyngitis, voice alteration, headache, dyspepsia, nasal congestion, and oral candidiasis. Rinsing the mouth with water after use will help minimize dry mouth, hoarseness, and oral candidiasis.

Wetting Agents

Medication	Dosage	Indications/Actions	Contraindications/Notes
water sterile, distilled	Intermittent or continuous nebulization	**Thick Secretions** *Humidify/thin/liquefy secretions* *Diluent of drugs*	Potential mucosal irritation, over-hydration, bronchospasm
Saline: Hypotonic (0.45% NaCl)			Same as above Less irritating than H_2O
Saline: Isotonic (0.9%)			Bronchospasm
Saline: Hypertonic	**Aerosol:** intermittent only (2-5 mL)	**Sputum Induction** *Above + osmotic transudat.*	Bronchospasm, mucosal irritation, edema, ↑blood Na+

Combination: Corticosteroid and LABA

Medication	Dosage	Summary of Action	Contraindications/Notes
budesonide and formoterol *Symbicort*	Inhalation ≥ 5 yrs 80mcg budesonide/ 4.5 formoterol 2 inhalations 2x/day Inhalation: 160 mcg budesonide/ 4.5 mcg formoterol 2 inhalations 2x/day	Long-term maintenance treatment of asthma in persons over 12 years old, who are not easily controlled with corticosteroid and occassional use of a SABA. *Combines action of systemic corti- costeroid and LABA*	**SEE BLACK BOX WARNING** SYMBICORT: Instruct patients to shake inhaler for a full 5 seconds prior to using, to mix medications. Rinse mouth after use Adverse: sore nose/throat, head- ache, stomach irritation, sinusitis, cardiovascular side effects
fluticasone and salmeterol *Advair*	DPI: 100/50, 250/50, 500/50 (fluticasone/salmeterol) Asthma (100/50, 250/50) COPD (250/50) 1 inhalation 2x/day, max 2/day HFA (LT maint.): (45/21, 115/21, 230/21) >12 yr: 2 inh. 2x/day, max 4/day	LT maintenance treatment of asthma in persons > 12 yrs Maintenance treatment (250/50) of airway obstruction associated with **Chronic Bronchitis**	Contraindicated as a rescue inhaler
See insert for recommended dosages for Asthma pts not adequately controlled by corticosteroids			

Combination: Corticosteroid and LABA

Medication	Dosage	Summary of Action	Contraindications/Notes
mometasone and formoterol	INHALATION 100 mcg/5 mcg 200 mcg/5 mcg ≥ 12 yrs: 2 inhalations, 2x/day Max 4 inhalations/day	Long term maintenance treatment of asthma	SEE BLACK BOX WARNING
Dulera			Same as Above

Combination: Anti-Cholinergic and SABA

Medication	Dosage	Indications/Actions	Contraindications/Notes
ipratropium bromide and albuterol	AEROSOL (0.5 mg ipratropium/ 2.5 mg albuterol) 3 mL nebulized 4x/day, with 2 additional doses if needed	COPD with bronchospasm	Do not administered with sympathomimetics/MAO inhibitors
Duoneb		*SABA and anticholinergic combined effects, which are thought to have a greater effect than either drug independently*	Paradoxical Bronchospasm
ipratropium bromide and albuterol	MDI: 18 mcg ipratropium bromide and 103 mcg albuterol sulfate		Caution with glaucoma, prostatic hypertrophy
Combivent	2 inhalations 4x/day, not to exceed 12 inhalations a day		

Combination: Anticholinergic and LABA

Medication	Dosage	Indications/Actions	Contraindications/Notes
umeclidinium and vilanterol *Anoro Ellipta*	62.5 mcg/25 mcg per puff 1 inhalations, once daily	**COPD long-term maintenance** *LABA and anticholinergic combined effects, which are thought to have a greater effect than either drug independently*	See Black Box Warning on pg 12-13 Do not use for acute symptoms
glycopyrrolate and formoterol *Bevespi Aerosphere*	9 mcg/4.8 mcg per puff steady state = 2-3 days 2 inhalations, 2x/day		Not indicated for Asthma
tiotropium and olodaterol *Stiolto Respimat*	3.1 mcg/2.7 mcg per puff (equiv to 2.5/2.5 mcg) 2 inhalations, once daily		
glycopyrrolate and indacaterol *Utibron Neohaler*	27.5 mcg/15.6 mcg per cap Inhale 1 cap every 12 hrs via Neohaler		

Medications Affecting Ventilation

Drugs that Cause Respiratory Depression

Ethyl alcohol

Hallucinogens (PCP, angel dust)

Narcotics: codeine, heroin, propoxyphene (Darvon), oxycodone (Percodan), fentanyl (Sublimaze),hydromorphone (Dialaudid), meperidine (Demerol), morphine

Sedatives/Hypnotics:

chloral hydrate, diazepam (Valium), lorazepam (Ativan), midazolan (Versed), zolpidem (Ambien)

Barbiturates:

phenobarbital, pentobarbital, thiopental (Pentothal)

Anesthetics: Propofol (Diprivan)

Paralytics (should not be administered without appropriate sedation, pt will cease ventilatory effort, airway must be managed). Several popular drugs, some of which have reversal agents (notable exception: succinylchonine, or "succs")

Drugs that Cause Respiratory Stimulation

Acids (CO_2, HCl, NH3Cl)

Adrenergic agents: ampheamine, ephedrine, norepinephrine

Alcohol: ethylene glycol (antifreeze)

Analeptics: doxapram (Dopram)

Benzodiazepine antagonists: flumazenil (Romazicon)

Diuretics: carbonic anhydrase inhibitors: acetazolamide

Hormones: ACTH, estrogen, insulin, progesterone, thyroxine

Irritants: ammonia, ether

Narcotic antagonist: naloxone (Narcan)

Salicylates: aspirin

Xanthines: aminophylline, caffeine, theophylline

See Oakes' Ventilator Management for detailed information on Critical Care Drugs, inlcuding Diuretics, Anticoagulants, Paralytics and Paralytic-Reversal Drugs

Oakes'
Ventilator
Management
An Oakes Pocket Guide

Dana Oakes
Sean Shortall

Common Cardiovascular Drugs

Anti-Arrhythmics

adenosine (Adenocard)	mexiletine
amiodarone	phenytoin (Dilantin)
diltiazem (Cardizem)	procainamide
disopyramide	(Procan, Pronestyl)
doletilide	propafenone (Rhythmol)
esmolol	propranolol (Inderal)
fosphenytoin (Cerebyx)	quinidine (Cardoquin)
ibutilide (Corvert)	tocainide (Tonocard)
lidocaine (Xylocaine)	verapamil (Calan, Isoptin)

Vasodilators (Vessel Dilation)

captopril (Capoten)	nicardipine (Cardene)
enalapril (Vasotec)	nitroglycerin
fenoldopam (Corlopam)	phentolamine (Regitime)
isoproterenol (Isuprel)	sodium nitroprusside
hydralazine (Apresoline)	(Nipride, Nitropress)
labetalol (Nomodyne, Trandate)	tolazoline (Priscoline)
nesiritide	

Inotropics (↑ Cardiac Contractility)

amrinone (Inocor)	epinephrine (Adrenalin)
digoxin (Lanoxin)	isoproterenol (Isuprel)
dobutamine (Dobutrex)	milrinone (Primacor)
dopamine (Intropin)	

Vasopressors (Vessel Constriction)

ephedrine (Bofedrol, Ephed)	norepinephrine or levartere-
metaraminol bitartrate	nol (Levophed)
(Aramine)	phenylephrine (Neosynephrine)

See Oakes' Hemodynamic Monitoring for expanded information on Cardiovascular Physiology

PHARM

13   Resuscitation

CONTENTS

CPR

This Chapter is a Summary of the *2015 American Heart Association* Guidelines for Cardiopulmonary Resuscitation and Emergency Cardiovascular Care Science

Basic Life Support (In Hospital) Algorithm

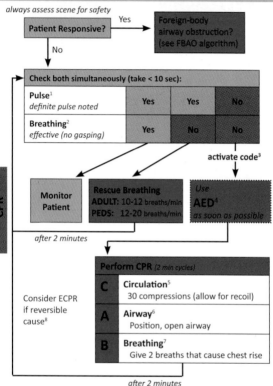

Minimize Interruptions at all stages -
continuous, high quality chest compressions are a priority.

FOOTNOTES
(see also Summarized CPR Components)
(see supporting figures on pg 13-5 to 13-7)

1- Check Pulse - Take no less than 5, but no more than 10 sec
Adult/child: use carotid or femoral
Infant < 1 yr: use brachial

2- Check Breathing - Simultaneously check breathing with pulse. Note that gasping/agonal breathing is NOT effective breathing.

3- Witnessed Collapse: Call code or send someone for help immediately
Unwitnessed Collapse in Peds: Give 2 mins CPR, then seek help/AED
in Adults: Call code or send someone for help

4- AED: Focus is on use as early as possible but with minimal interruption to chest compressions. **SEE PG 13-8 for in-depth AED info.**

5- Chest Compressions - Equal compression/relaxation ratio. Avoid leaning on chest during relaxation phase (may restrict recoil)
See figures 12-17 on pg 13-6
  2 Rescuers:
  Unsecured airway - Pause compressions for ventilations. Begin compressions at peak inspiration of 2nd breath.
  Secured airway - Do not pause or synchronize for ventilations. Change roles every 2 mins to avoid tiring (↓ quality of compressions)

6- Open Airway -
  Head tilt - **chin lift**: preferred when no evidence of head or neck trauma. See figure 1 on pg 13-5
  Jaw thrust: See figure 2 on pg 13-5
        Primarily for C-Spine caution (do not tilt head)
        Open mouth and remove any visible foreign material, vomitus, or loose dentures (Fig 20). Blind finger sweeps are not indicated.

7- Provide Breathing - Avoid large, rapid or forceful breaths. Do not deliver more volume or force than is needed to produce visible chest rise. Use mouth to mouth/nose for infants (See ACLS Section)
See figures 4-12 on pg 13-5 and 13-6

8- ECPR. Extracorporeal CPR (initiation of extracorporeal circulation and oxygenation during resuscitation). The goal is to support pts in arrest while treating reversible conditions. Studies have focused on 18-75 yrs.

CPR Components, Summarized
(Infant, Child, Adult)

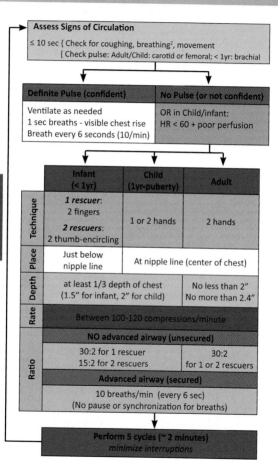

Assess Signs of Circulation

≤ 10 sec { Check for coughing, breathing[2], movement
{ Check pulse: Adult/Child: carotid or femoral; < 1yr: brachial

Definite Pulse (confident)	No Pulse (or not confident)
Ventilate as needed 1 sec breaths - visible chest rise Breath every 6 seconds (10/min)	OR in Child/infant: HR < 60 + poor perfusion

		Infant (< 1yr)	Child (1yr-puberty)	Adult
	Technique	**1 rescuer:** 2 fingers **2 rescuers:** 2 thumb-encircling	1 or 2 hands	2 hands
	Place	Just below nipple line	At nipple line (center of chest)	
	Depth	at least 1/3 depth of chest (1.5" for infant, 2" for child)		No less than 2" No more than 2.4"
	Rate	Between 100-120 compressions/minute		
	Ratio	**NO advanced airway (unsecured)**		
		30:2 for 1 rescuer 15:2 for 2 rescuers		30:2 for 1 or 2 rescuers
		Advanced airway (secured)		
		10 breaths/min (every 6 sec) (No pause or synchronization for breaths)		

Perform 5 cycles (~ 2 minutes)
minimize interruptions

13-4

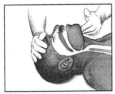

Fig. 1. Head tilt-chin lift

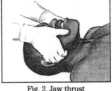

Fig. 2. Jaw thrust
(without head tilt)

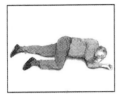

Fig. 3. Recovery position

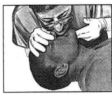

Fig. 4. Mouth-to-mouth
rescue breathing

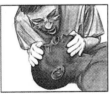

Fig. 5. Mouth-to-nose
rescue breathing

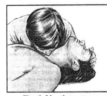

Fig. 6. Mouth-to-stoma
rescue breathing

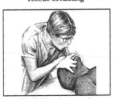

Fig. 7. Mouth-to-mask
cephalic technique

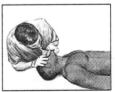

Fig. 8. Mouth-to-mask
lateral technique

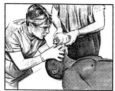

Fig. 9. Two rescuer use
of the bag mask

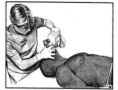

Fig. 10. One rescuer use
of the bag mask

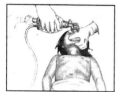

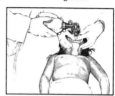

Fig. 11. Bag-mask ventilation for child victim
A, 1 rescuer; B, 2 rescuers

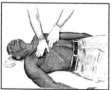

Fig. 12. Positioning of rescuer's
hands for chest compressions

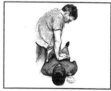

Fig. 13. Position of rescuer
for chest compressions

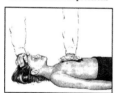

Fig. 14. One hand chest
compression in child

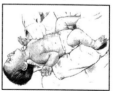

Fig. 15. One rescuer
infant CPR while carrying

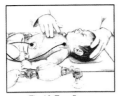

Fig. 16. Two finger
chest compression

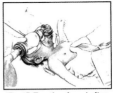

Fig. 17. Two thumb-encircling
hands chest compression

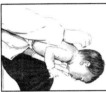

Fig. 18. Infant back blows

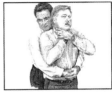

Fig. 19. Heimlich maneuver,
victim standing

Automatic External Defibrillator (AED)

Witnessed Arrest	Unwitnessed Arrest
Use AED ASAP	Initiate CPR Use AED as soon as device is ready

Rhythms (child and adult only):
- Shockable Rhythm:
  Give 1 shock, immediately resume CPR (beginning with compressions), do not check pulse. Recheck rhythm in 2 minutes.
- Not Shockable Rhythm:
  Immediately resume CPR. Recheck rhythm in 2 minutes.

Notes: Rescuers must practice minimizing the time between compressions to give a shock.

Infants (< 1 yr)

1st Preference:	Manual Defibrillator
2nd Preference:	AED with pediatric dose attenuator
3rd Preference	AED without a dose attenuator may be used if above two are not available

Children

1st Attempt	2 Joules/kg
Subsequent Attempts	at least 4 Joules/kg, *not to exceed 10 Joules/kg* *or the adult maximum dose*

Ages 1- 8 yrs
use pediatric dose-attenuator system, if available.

Opioid-Associated Life-Threatening Emergencies*

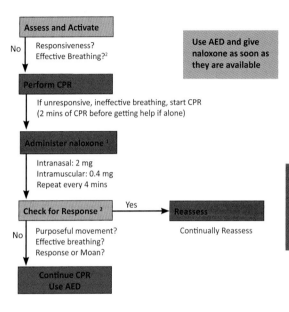

Assess and Activate

No | Responsiveness?
Effective Breathing?[2]

Use AED and give naloxone as soon as they are available

Perform CPR

If unresponsive, ineffective breathing, start CPR
(2 mins of CPR before getting help if alone)

Administer naloxone [1]

Intranasal: 2 mg
Intramuscular: 0.4 mg
Repeat every 4 mins

Check for Response [2] → Yes → **Reassess**

No | Purposeful movement?
Effective breathing?
Response or Moan?

Continually Reassess

**Continue CPR
Use AED**

CPR

---

* Summarized from AHA 2015 Guidelines
[1] Cardiac arrest is usually secondary to respiratory arrest with opioids
[2] Do not delay CPR to await response to naloxone

Foreign-Body Airway Obstruction (FBAO)

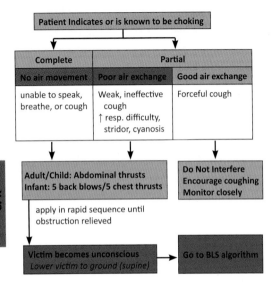

CPR

Complete	Partial	
No air movement	Poor air exchange	Good air exchange
unable to speak, breathe, or cough	Weak, ineffective cough ↑ resp. difficulty, stridor, cyanosis	Forceful cough

Patient Indicates or is known to be choking

Adult/Child: Abdominal thrusts
Infant: 5 back blows/5 chest thrusts

apply in rapid sequence until obstruction relieved

Do Not Interfere
Encourage coughing
Monitor closely

Victim becomes unconscious
Lower victim to ground (supine)

Go to BLS algorithm

Notes:
Infant/child –
5 Back blows/5 Chest thrusts: one every sec as needed, same location and technique as chest compressions
Abdominal thrusts not recommended for infants (<1 yr)
Sudden respiratory distress (coughing, gagging, and/or stridor) accompanied by fever, congestion, hoarseness, drooling or lethargy are indicative of infections such as epiglottitis or croup. The child must be taken immediately to an emergency facility because back blows or chest thrusts will not relieve the obstruction.
Late pregnancy – use chest thrusts
Obesity – use chest thrusts (if rescuer cannot encircle abdomen)

ACLS/PALS

Airways

Adjuncts

Oropharyngeal Airway	• Use only in unconscious (unresponsive) patients with no cough or gag reflex. • Should be inserted only by trained personnel. • Note: Incorrect insertion can displace the tongue into hypopharynx.
Nasopharyngeal Airway	• Useful in patients with (or at risk of developing) airway obstruction (particularly clenched jaw). • May be better tolerated than oropharyngeal in patients not deeply unconscious. • Caution in patients with severe cranial facial injury. • May be easily obstructed by secretions in infants

CPR

Advanced Airways (General)	
Advantages	• Isolation of airway • Reduced risk of aspiration • Potentially improved ventilation and oxygenation • Allows CPR without interruption of compressions • Ability to use capnography to monitor quality of CPR, optimize chest compressions, and detect ROSC during chest compressions
Disadvantages	• Insertion may require interruption of chest compressions. • May defer insertion until patient fails to respond to initial CPR or demonstrates ROSC. • Risk of unrecognized esophageal intubation
Notes	• Optimal method (bag-mask, ET tube, Combitube, or LMA) depends on rescuer experience, patient's condition, and system. • Healthcare providers must maintain knowledge and skills through frequent practice with these devices. • Once advanced airway is in place, 2 rescuers no longer deliver cycles of CPR. • Infants and children: In out-of-hospital setting, bag and mask ventilation preferred over intubation, if transport is short.

CPR

Endotracheal (ET) Tube

Indications	• Inability to ventilate unconscious patient with bag and mask • Absence of airway protective reflexes (coma, cardiac arrest)
Advantages	• Patent airway • Drug administration • High Oxygen delivery route • Specific VT delivery • Cuff protection • Permits suctioning
Technique	• Inserter must be trained and experienced. • Minimize the number and duration of interruptions to chest compressions (be fully prepared to insert when compressing rescuer pauses) to < 10 seconds. Compressions should resume as soon as the tube passes through the vocal cords. Provide adequate ventilation/compressions between attempts. • Pulse oximetry and ECG should be monitored continuously during intubation of patient with a perfusing rhythm. Interrupt attempt if oxygenation/ventilation is needed.
Verify Placement	• Auscultation: BS equal/bilateral, BS absent over epigastrum • Chest expansion • ETCO$_2$ detector or EDD (see 10-24) • Continuous waveform capnography is recommended • SpO$_2$ only if a perfusing rhythm
Notes	• No one single confirmation technique is completely reliable (including H$_2$O vapor). If any doubt: Use larynogoscope to visualize tube passing through vocal cords. If still doubt, remove tube. • Remove tube at once if hear stomach gurgling and see no chest expansion. • Children: Body Length is most reliable (use tape), but **in emergency use:**

	Uncuffed Tube	Cuffed Tube
< 1 yr	3.5 mm ID	3.0 mm ID
1-2 yrs	4.0 mm ID	3.5 mm ID
> 2 yrs	3.5 + (age/4)	3.5 + (age/4)

Notes	• If an intubated pt's condition deteriorates, consider the following (DOPE):
	  • **D**isplacement of the tube
	  • **O**bstruction of the tube
	  • **P**neumothorax
	  • **E**quipment failure

Alternatives	• Laryngeal Mask Airway (LMA). May be advantageous when access to pt is limited, presence of unstable neck injury, or positioning for intubation impossible • Esophageal-tracheal tube (Combitube): confirmation of placement is essential

See Bag-Mask Ventilation on page 10-24.

Considerations / Notes	
Cricoid Pressure	• Is not routinely recommended • May help prevent gastric inflation. • Use only if victim is deeply unconscious (no cough or gag reflex). • Usually requires third rescuer
Regurgitation	• If patient vomits, turn to side, wipe out mouth, return to supine, and continue CPR

Capnography/ Capnometry	• Continuous quantitative waveform capnography is recommended for intubated patients through the peri-arrest period for:
	• Confirming tracheal tube placement
	• Monitoring CPR quality and therapy
	• Detecting ROSC based upon end-tidal carbon dioxide ($PetCO_2$) values
	  • If $PetCO_2$ <10 mm Hg, attempt to improve CPR quality
	  • An abrupt and sustained rise in $PetCO_2$ may be observed just before clinical identification of ROSC, so use of $PetCO_2$ monitoring may reduce the need to interrupt chest compressions for a pulse check.
	  • Falling cardiac output or rearrest in the patient with ROSC causes a decrease in $PetCO_2$.

CPR

Monitoring	
Pulses	• Take < 10 sec to palpate for pulse; resume compressions immediately in unable to feel. • Carotid pulsations during CPR do not indicate the efficacy of coronary, myocardial or cerebral perfusion. Femoral pulsations may indicate venous rather than arterial flow • If A-line monitor: maximize BP dia (ideally ≥30 − 10 = 20 mmHg)
Oximetry	• During arrest, SpO_2 is a poor indicator • Upon ROSC, use SpO2 to titrate inspired Oxygen (when equipment available) - maintain an SaO2 ≥ 94%, but < 100% to limit the risk of hyperoxemia. • $ScvO_2$: Indicator of CO and O_2 delivery during CPR. If CVP line in place, can you monitor CPR effectiveness (should be > 30%) and detect ROSC without interrupting chest compressions to check rhythm and pulse.
ABG's	Not a reliable indicator of the severity of tissue hypoxemia, hypercarbia (ie., ventilation), or tissue acidosis during arrest
$ETCO_2$	• Safe and effective indicator of CO (+ may be ROSC) during CPR • If ventilation is reasonably constant: $\Delta CO_2 ≈ \Delta CO$ • An abrupt sustained increase in $PETCO_2$ during CPR is an indicator of ROSC. • A transient rise in $PETCO_2$ after sodium bicarbonate therapy is expected and should not be misinterpreted as an improvement in quality of CPR or a sign of ROSC. • Persistently low $PETCO_2$ values (< 10 mm Hg) during CPR in intubated pts suggest that ROSC is unlikely. • Monitoring $PETCO_2$ trends during CPR has the potential to guide individual optimization of compression depth and rate and to detect fatigue in the provider performing compressions. • After CPR – use to guide ventil. (along w/ ABG) + ET tube position

Post-Resuscitation Care

Recommendations
1. Optimize cardiopulmonary function and vital organ perfusion after ROSC
2. Transport/transfer to an appropriate hospital or critical care unit with a comprehensive post–cardiac arrest treatment system of care
3. Identify and treat ACS and other reversible causes

H's	T's
Hypoxia	Toxins
Hypovolemia	Trauma
Hyperthermia	Thrombosis
Hypoglycemia	Tamponade (cardiac)
Hypo/hyperkalemia	Tension pneumothorax
Hydrogen ion (acidosis)	Treat consequences (hypoxia, ischemia, reperfusion)

4. Targeted Temperature Management: Comatose pts should be kept at a target temp of 34-36°C for 24+ hrs after Return of Spontaneous Circulation (ROSC). Preventing fever after 24 hours is an indication for continuing a hypothermic state.
5. Anticipate, treat, and prevent multiple organ dysfunction. This includes avoiding excessive ventilation and hyperoxia

Withdrawal of Support

Be cautious about determination of poor neurological outcome when using hypothermia (targeted temperature management) protocols, presence of shock, or when sedation is used.
Poor neurological outcome is supported by:
- Absent pupillary response at 24 hrs
- Persistent absence of EEG reactivity to external stimuli at 72 hrs
- CT/MRI confirmation may be quicker
- Absence of movement and posturing should NOT be used independently for predicting outcomes

Post-Cardiac Arrest Care

Ventilation	
Capnography	• Confirm secure airway and titrate ventilation • ET Tube when possible for comatose patients • $PETCO_2 \approx 35{-}40$ mm Hg • $PaCO_2 \approx 40{-}45$ mm Hg
CXR	Confirm secure airway and detect causes or complications of arrest: pneumonitis, pneumonia, pulmonary edema

Pulse Oximetry/ ABG	• Maintain adequate oxygenation and minimize FIO_2
	  • $SpO_2 \geq 94\%$
	  • $PaO_2 \approx 100$ mmHg
	• Reduce FIO_2 as tolerated
	• PaO_2/FIO_2 ratio to follow acute lung injury

Mechanical Ventilation	• Minimize acute lung injury, potential oxygen toxicity
	• Tidal Volume 6–8 mL/kg
	• Titrate minute ventilation to
	  • $PETCO_2 \approx 35{-}40$ mm Hg
	  • $PaCO_2 \approx 40{-}45$ mm Hg
	• Avoid hyperventilation *
	• Reduce FiO_2 as tolerated to keep SpO_2 or SaO2 ≥94%

* Achieve normocarbia – avoid hyperventilation
After ROSC, there is commonly a brief period (10-30 min) of cerebral hyperemia, followed by a prolonged period of hyporemia.
Potential detrimental effects of hyperventilation:
   ↑ PIT → ↓CO → ↓cerebral blood flow → ↑ ischemia
   ↓PCO2 → cerebral vasoconstriction → ↓cerebral blood flow → ↑ ischemia
   ↑ Paw and/or ↑ auto-PEEP → ↑ intracranial pressure, → ↓cerebral blood flow → ↑ ischemia

CPR

Hemodynamics	
Freq BP Monitoring/ A-Line	• Maintain perfusion and prevent recurrent hypotension • Mean Arterial Pressure ≥65 mm Hg or systolic blood pressure ≥ 90 mm Hg
Treat Hypotension	Maintain perfusion; Fluid bolus if tolerated Dopamine 5–10 mcg/kg per min Norepinephrine 0.1–0.5 mcg/kg per min Epinephrine 0.1–0.5 mcg/kg per min

Cardiovascular
Continuous Cardiac Monitoring
12-lead ECG/Troponin, Echocardiogram
Treat Myocardial Stunning and Acute Coronary Syndrome

Neurological	
Serial Neuro Exam	• Define coma, brain injury, and prognosis • Response to verbal commands or physical stimulation • Pupillary light and coronary reflex, spont eye movement • Gag, cough, spontaneous breaths
EEG Monitoring if Coma	• Exclude seizures • Anticonvulsants if seizing
Sedation/ Muscle Relaxation	• To control shivering, agitation, or ventilator dyssynchrony as needed

Metabolic	
Serial Lactate	• Confirm adequate perfusion
Serum Potassium	• Avoid hypokalemia which promotes arrhythmias • Replace to maintain K > 3.5 mEq/L

Urine Output, Serum Creatinine
Serum Glucose
Avoid Hypotonic Fluid

CPR

13-18

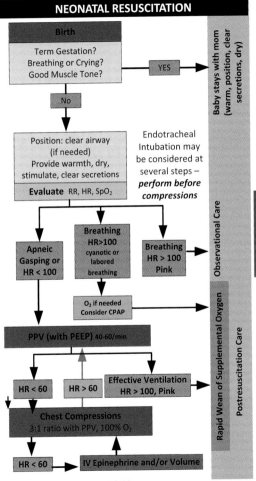

NEONATAL RESUSCITATION

Birth

Term Gestation?
Breathing or Crying?
Good Muscle Tone?

YES → Baby stays with mom (warm, position, clear secretions, dry)

No

Position: clear airway (if needed)
Provide warmth, dry, stimulate, clear secretions

Evaluate RR, HR, SpO₂

Endotracheal Intubation may be considered at several steps – *perform before compressions*

Apneic Gasping or HR < 100

Breathing HR>100 cyanotic or labored breathing

Breathing HR > 100 Pink

O₂ if needed
Consider CPAP

PPV (with PEEP) 40-60/min

HR < 60   **HR > 60**   **Effective Ventilation HR > 100, Pink**

Chest Compressions
3:1 ratio with PPV, 100% O₂

HR < 60 → **IV Epinephrine and/or Volume**

Observational Care

CPR

Rapid Wean of Supplemental Oxygen

Postresuscitation Care

13-19

Targeted Preductal SpO$_2$ after Birth

Oxygen administration should be guided by SpO$_2$ (pulse oximeter on upper right extremity - such as wrist or palm)

Time	Target SpO$_2$
1 minute	60-65%
2 minutes	65-70%
3 minutes	70-75%
4 minutes	75-80%
5 minutes	80-85%
10 minutes	85-95%

The following pages are summarized from the American Heart Association Neonatal Resusictation Program, published November, 2015.

Summary of Neonatal Resuscitation Guidelines:

1. **Preparation and Team Briefing**
2. **Initial Steps**
3. **Use of Positive-Pressure Ventilation (PPV)**
4. **Chest Compressions**
5. **Drugs Administered**
6. **Post-Resuscitation Care**
7. **Ethics / Discontinuation**

1. Preparation and Team Briefing

- Verify that all supplies are available and that equipment is functional.
- Every birth should be attended by at least 1 person who can perform resuscitation.
- Every high-risk birth should be attended by a team of people who can perform resuscitation, with a team leader identified, and a briefing performed.

2. Initial Steps

> **Body temperature goal:** 36.5 - 37.5° C
> Dry/Stimulate
> Avoid routine suctioning
> Careful oxygen administration

- Neonatal body temperature should be maintained between 36.5 C- 37.5 C with no asphyxia, particularly in neonates < 32 wks gestation. Radiant warmers, plastic wrap, thermal mattresses, warmed humidified gases are all reasonable strategies. NOTE that hyperthermia is a risk.
- <u>Routine</u> suctioning (bulb syringe or catheter) is not recommended, regardless of presence of meconium-stained amniotic fluid. Greatest emphasis is on initiating ventilation within 1st minute of life.

- Heart rate can best be monitored using a 3-lead ECG, while oxygenation can be best monitored using pulse oximetry. Increase in HR is seen as a very sensitive measure of success in resuscitation efforts.
- Oxygen administration should be maintained within a safe range (no hypoxia, no hyperoxia). Use targeted ranges on pg 1-4.
  - ≥ 35 wks: Start with Room Air (RA)
  - < 35 wks: Start with 21-30%
  - If SpO_2 is not in target range, start with 30% (free-flow @ 10 L/min). If SpO_2 is still below range and on 100%, trial CPAP. If baby is not breathing, use PPV (below).

3. Use of Positive-Pressure Ventilation (PPV)

> **Manually ventilate** 40-60 breaths/min
> **Use CPAP/PEEP** with pre-term neonates

Manual Resuscitation
- Rates of 40-60 breaths/min are most common.
- Increase of HR > 100/min is best indicator of success
- Use enough pressure to see gentle rise of chest.
- Start with 5-6 cmH_2O PEEP in preterm neonates.
- Auscultate HR (over heart) for 1st 15 seconds - you are checking for an increasing HR.
- Understand how to properly use the type of resuscitator available in your delivery room.
- If < 30 wks, consider having surfactant ready

Intubation
- Consider intubating when unable to ventilate effectively, or no improvement with BVM, when compressions are performed, and in unique situations (Congenital Diaphragmatic Hernia, for example) .
- Exhaled CO_2 is recommended method of confirming ET Tube placement (except if perfusion is poor, such as cardiac arrest). Other methods include chest movement, breath sounds, and condensate in ET tube.

- Remember, vocal cord indicator on ET Tube is an estimation of placement, and should not be used to confirm placement.

4. Chest Compressions

> **Technique:** 2-thumb technique preferred
> **Depth:** ⅓ A-P diameter on lower 3rd of sternum
> **Rate:** 120 compressions/breaths per minute
> **Synchronize with compressions** (3:1 ratio)

- Compressions are indicated when HR < 60/min despite adequate ventilation.
- 100% O_2 is indicated during compressions (wean aggressively once HR recovers).
- Compressions should be delivered on lower third of sternum, with a depth of ~⅓ A-P diameter.
- 2-thumb technique is preferred method (do not use 2-finger technique).
- Coordinate compressions/ventilations at a ratio of 3:1 (120 events per minute) unless cardiac in origin (then use 15:2).
- RR, HR, SpO_2 should be reassessed periodically, but avoid frequent interruptions.

CPR

5. Drugs Administered

- Drug administration is uncommon as bradycardia is usually caused by ventilation issues/hypoxemia.
- The use of Epinephrine and/or Volume is indicated when HR < 60/min despite ventilation with 100% O_2 and chest compressions.

SEE DRUGS NEXT PAGE

Epinephrine

*Epinephrine is considered after PPV and compressions
have been trialed (see NRP algorithm).*

1:10 000 Epinephrine by IV:
   0.1 - 0.3 mL/kg

1:10 000 Epinephrine by ET Tube:
   0.3 - 1 mL/kg

1:10 000 Epinephrine ≈ 0.1 mg/mL

Volume Expansion

*Volume expansion is considered when blood loss is known
or suspected, HR has not responded otherwise. Early
administration increases risk of IVH.*

Isotonic Crystalloid Solution   or
Blood

10 mL/kg/dose

CPR

6. Post-Resuscitation Care
- IV glucose infusion should be considered to avoid hypo-glycemia (hypoglycemia increases risk of brain injury).
- Therapeutic Hypothermia should be considered with moderate-severe hypoxic-ischemic encephalopathy.

7. Ethics / Discontinuation
- If it is believed there is no chance for survival, resuscita-tion should not be offered.
- If there is a questionable risk for survival, parents should be included in the decision-making process regarding resuscitation efforts.

A Appendix

CONTENTS

Symbols

Basic Units of Measure

cmH₂0	centimeters of water pressure		
°C	degrees of temperature in centigrade	sec	seconds
ft	foot	m	meters
gm%	gram percent (number of grams per 100 grams of total weight)	vol%	volume percent (number of mL of a substance per 100 mL of total volume)
in.	inch	beats/min(bpm)	heart beats per minute
kcal	kilocalorie	breaths/min	breaths per minute
kg	kilograms	L/min	liters per minute
kPa	SI unit for pressure*	L/sec	liters per second
l or L	liters	mEq/L	milliequivalents per liter
L/kPa	SI unti for compliance*	mg/mL	milligrams per milliliter
mL	milliliters	mL/min	milliliters per minute
min	minutes	mL/kg	milliliters per kilogram
mM	millimole	SI	standard international unit*
mmHg	millimeters of mercury pressure		

SI equivalents: kPa=mmHg x 0.133   L/kPa=L/cmH2O x 10.2   kPa=cmH2O x 0.098

Basic Gas Phase Symbols

Primary Symbols

D	diffusion	R	respiratory exchange ratio
F	fractional concentration of a gas	V	volume of gas
P	partial pressure of a gas	$\dot{V}$	flow of gas (volume/time)
$\overline{P}$	mean pressure of a gas		

Qualifying Subscripts

anat	anatomic	E	expired	BTPS	body conditions: body temperature and ambient pressure, saturated with water vapor at these conditions
aw	airway	I	inspired		
dyn	dynamic	L	lung		
eso	esophagus	S	static		
f	frequency	T	tidal	ATPD	ambient temp and press, dry
phy	physiologic	CO2	carbon dioxide	ATPS	ambient temperature and pressure, saturated with water vapor at these conditions
pl	pleural	O2	oxygen		
stat	static	N2	nitrogen		
t	time	H20	water	STPD	standard conditions: temperature 0°C, pressure 760 torr, and dry (0 torr water vapor)
A(alv)	alveolar				
B	barometric				
D	deadspace				

Basic Blood Phase Symbols

Primary Symbols	Qualifying Subscripts
Q volume of blood	a arterial
Q̇ blood flow (cardiac output), L/min	c capillary
C concentation (content in the blood phase)	c pulmonary end - capillary
	s shunt
S saturation in the blood phase	v venous
	v̄ mixed venous

A-2

Abbreviations

Abbr.	Definition	Abbr.	Definition	Abbr.	Definition	Abbr.	Definition
AARC	American Association of Respiratory Care	bpm	Beats or breaths/minute	COPD	Chronic obstructive pulmonary disease	ECG	Electrocardiogram
ABG	Arterial blood gas	BPsys	Systolic blood pressure	CPAP	Continuous positive airway pressure	ECMO	Extracorporeal membrane oxygenation
A/C	Assist/control	B-P	Broncho-pleural	CPG	Clinical Practice Guideline	EDV	End diastolic volume
ACCP	American College of Chest Physicians	BSA	Body surface area	CPP	Cerebral or coronary perfusion pressure	EEP	End expiratory pressure
ACLS	Advanced Cardiac Life Support	CABG	Coronary artery bypass graph	CPR	Cardio-pulmonary resuscitation	EGTA	Esophageal-gastric tube airway
ADH	Anti-diuretic hormone	CaO_2	Arterial oxygen content	CPT	Chest physical therapy	EKG	Electrocardiogram
A-fib	Atrial fibrillation	$Ca-\bar{v}O_2$	Arterial –mixed venous O_2 content difference	CSF	Cerebral spinal fluid	EPAP	Expiratory positive airway pressure
AG	Anion gap	CB	Chronic Bronchitis	Cstat	Static compliance	ERV	Expiratory reserve volume
AHA	American Heart Assoc	CC	Closing capacity	Ctubing	Compliance of the tubing	et	End-tidal
ALI	Acute lung injury	Ccw	Chest wall compliance	CV	Cardiovascular	ET	Endotracheal
AMI	Acute Myocardial infarct	CHD	Congenital heart disease	CVA	Cerebrovascular accident	ETS	Endotracheal suction
A-P	Anterior-Posterior	CHF	Congestive heart failure	CvO_2	Venous oxygen content	EIA	Exercise induced asthma
ARDS	Acute respiratory distress syndrome	Cdyn	Dynamic compliance	CVP	Central venous pressure	f	Frequency (ventilator rate)
ARF	Acute respiratory failure	CF	Conversion factor/Cystic Fibrosis	CXR	Chest x-ray	FDO_2	Fraction of delivered O_2
ASD	Atrial septal defect	CI	Cardiac index	D	Deadspace or diffusion	$FECO_2$	Fractional concentration of expired CO_2
AV	Atrio-ventricular	CL	Compliance of the lung	DKA	Diabetic ketoacidosis	FEF	Forced expiratory flow
a-v	arterio-venous	CLT	Compliance of the lung and thorax	DLCO	Diffusion capacity for CO	FEV	Forced expiratory volume
BE/BD	Base excess/deficit	cm H2O	Centimeters of water	DO_2	Oxygen delivery	FICO	Fraction of inspired CO
BiPAP	Bi-level positive airway pressure	CMV	Cytomegaly virus	DOE	Dyspnea on exertion	FIF	Forced inspiratory flow
BLS	Basic Life Support	CNS	Central nervous system	DPG,2,3	2,3 diphosphoglycerate	FIO_2	Fraction of inspired oxygen
BP	Blood pressure	CO	Cardiac output	DPI	Dry powder inhaler	FIVC	Forced inspiratory vital capacity
BPdia	Diastolic blood pressure	CO	Carbon monoxide	E	Expiration	Fr	French
		CO_2	Carbon dioxide	ECC	Emergency cardiac care		

Abbreviation	Definition
FRC	Functional residual capacity
F-T	Flow-time
FVC	Forced vital capacity
Gaw	Airway conductance
GI	Gastrointestinal
H+	Hydrogen ion
HbO2	Oxyhemoglobin
HCH	Hygroscopic condenser humidifier
HCO3	Bicarbonate
Hct	Hematocrit
HFV	High frequency ventilation
Hgb	Hemoglobin
HME	Heat moisture exchanger
HR	Heart rate or heated reservoir
I	Inspiration
IC	Inspiratory capacity
ICP	Intracranial pressure
ID	Internal diameter
I:E	Inspiratory/expiratory ratio
IPAP	Inspiratory positive airway pressure
IMV	Intermittent mandatory ventilation
IO	Intraosseous
I+O	Intake & output
IPPV	Intermittent positive pressure breathing
IRV	Inspiratory reserve volume or Inverse ratio ventilation
IS	Incentive spirometry
IV	Intravenous
J	Joule
JVD	Jugular vein distention
kg	Kilogram
LA	Left atrium
LAP	Left atrial pressure
LDH	Lactic dehydrogenase
LOC	Level of consciousness
L-R	Left to right
LV	Left ventricle
LHF	Left heart failure
LVF	Left ventricular failure
LVH	Left ventricular hypertrophy
LVEDP	Left ventricular end diastolic pressure
LVEDV	Left ventricular end diastolic volume
LVESP	Left ventricular end systolic pressure
LVESV	Left ventricular end systolic volume
LVSW	Left ventricular stroke work
LVSWI	Left ventricular stroke work index
MAP	Mean arterial pressure
MBC	Maximum breathing capacity
MDI	Metered dose inhaler
MDO2	Myocardial oxygen delivery
MEF	Maximal expiratory pressure
MEFV	Maximal expiratory flow volume
MI	Myocardial infarction
MIF	See Pimax
MIP	See Pimax
mm Hg	millimeters of mercury
MvO2	Myocardial O2 consumption
MV	Mechanical ventilation
MVV	Maximum voluntary ventilation
NG	Nasogastric
NIF	See Pimax
N-M	Neuromuscular
NO	Nitric oxide
NPPV	Noninvasive positive pressure ventilation
NSS	Normal saline solution
NTS	Nasotracheal suction
O2	Oxygen
O2ER	Oxygen extraction ratio
O2 Sat	Oxygen saturation
P	Pressure
PA	Pulmonary artery or posterior-anterior
PA-aO2	Alveolar-arterial oxygen partial pressure difference
PaCO2	Partial pressure of arterial carbon dioxide
PACO2	Partial pressure of alveolar carbon dioxide
PAC	Premature atrial contraction
P-ACV	Pressure-assist/control ventilation
PAPD	Pulmonary artery diastolic pressure
PAEPD	Pulmonary artery end-diastolic pressure
Palv	Alveolar pressure
PAMP	Pulmonary artery mean pressure
PaO2	Partial pressure of arterial oxygen
PAO2	Partial pressure of alveolar oxygen
PAOP	Pulmonary artery occlusion pressure
PAP	Pulmonary artery pressure
PASP	Pulmonary artery systolic pressure
PAT	Premature atrial tachycardia
Paw	Airway pressure
$\overline{Paw}$	Mean airway pressure
Pawo	Pressure at airway opening

Abbreviation	Definition
PAWP	Pulmonary artery wedge pressure
PB	Barometric pressure
PBW	Predicted body weight
PCWP	Pulmonary capillary wedge pressure
Pcyl	Pressure in a cylinder
PDT	Postural drainage therapy
PEA	Pulseless electrical activity
PECO2	Partial pressure of expired CO_2
PetCO2	Partial pressure of end-expired CO_2
PEEP	Positive end-expiratory pressure
PEF	Peak expiratory flow
PEP	Positive expiratory pressure
PFT	Pulmonary function test
pH	Negative log of hydrogen ion concentration
pHa	pH of arterial blood
pHv	pH of venous blood
PIF	Peak inspiratory flow
PImax	Maximal inspiratory pressure
PIO2	Partial pressure of inspired O_2
PIP	Peak inspiratory pressure
PIT	Intrathoracic pressure
PIV	Intravascular pressure
PMI	Point of maximal impulse
PNC	Premature nodal contraction
PND	Paroxysmal nocturnal dyspnea
PP	Pulse pressure
PPE	Personal Protective Equipment
Ppl	Intrapleural pressure
Ppeak	Peak inspiratory pressure
Pplat	Inspiratory plateau pressure
PPV	Positive pressure ventilation
PSTV	Paroxysmal supra-ventricular tachycardia
PT	Prothrombin time
PtcO2	Transcutaneous partial pressure of oxygen
PTL	Pharyngo-tracheal lumen airway
Ptm	Transmural pressure
PTT	Partial prothrombin time
PV	Pressure ventilation
PVC	Premature ventricular contraction
PVD	Peripheral vascular disease
PTO2	Partial pressure of oxgen in mixed venous blood
PVR	Pulmonary vascular resistance
PVRI	Pulmonary vascular resistance index
P50	Pressure at 50% saturation
Q	Perfusion
Qc pul	Pulmonary capillary blood volume
Qpul	Pulmonary perfusion
Qs	Shunt
Qs anat	Anatomical shunt
Qs cap	Capillary shunt
Qs/Qt	Physiological shunt
QT	Total perfusion
R(RR)	Respiratory exchange ratio
Raw	Airway resistance
RA	Right atrium
RHF	Right heart failure
RAP	Right atrial pressure
RBC	Red blood cell
RFF	Ratio flow factor
RH	Right heart
RHF	Right heart failure
R-L	Right to left
ROSC	Return of spontaneous circulation
R pul	Pulmonary resistance
RQ	Respiratory quotient
RR	Spontaneous respiratory rate
RV	Right ventricle
RVEDP	Right ventricle end-diastolic pressure
RVEDV	Right ventricular end diastolic volume
RVESP	Right ventricular end systolic pressure
RVESV	Right ventricular end systolic volume
RVF	Right ventricular failure
RVSW	Right ventricular stroke work
RVSWI	Right ventricular stroke work index
SA	Sino-atrial
SaO2	Saturation of arterial oxygen
Sat	Saturation
SBN2	Single breath nitrogen washout
SCCM	Society of Critical Care Medicine
SMI	Sustained maximal inspiration
SOB	Shortness of breath
SPAG	Small particle aerosol generator
SpO2	Saturation of arterial oxygen

	by pulse oximeter	VC	Vital capacity
SV	Stroke volume	VCO2	Volume of carbon dioxide production
SVC	Slow vital capacity	VD	Deadspace volume
SVI	Stroke volume index	V̇D	Deadspace ventilation
SVN	Small volume nebulizer	VD anat	Anatomical deadspace
SVO2	Saturation of oxygen in mixed venous blood	VD mech	Mechanical deadspace
SVR	Systemic vascular resistance	VD phys	Physiological deadspace
SVRI	Systemic vascular resistance index	VD/VT	Deadspace/tidal volume ratio
SW	Stroke work	V̇E	Minute ventilation
SWI	Stroke work index	V̇Emech	Minute ventilation mechanical
TCO2	Total CO2	V̇Espont	Minute ventilation spontaneous
TDP	Therapist driven protocol	Vfib	Ventricular fibrillation
TE	Expiratory time	V̇I	Inspiratory flow
T-E	Tracheo-esophageal	VILI	Ventilator-induced lung injury
temp	Temperature	V̇O2	Volume of oxygen consumption
TF	Total flow	V-P	Volume-pressure (curve)
TI	Inspiratory time	VSD	Ventricular septal defect
TLC	Total lung capacity	VT	Tidal volume
Ttot	Total cycle time	Vtach	Ventricular tachycardia
UO	Urinary output	VTG	Thoracic gas volume
URI	Upper respiratory infection	Vtubing	Volume loss to tubing
USN	Ultrasonic nebulizer	V/Q	Ventilation/perfusion ratio
V̇	Volume or ventricular	VV	Volume ventilation
V̇	Flow		
v	Venous		
VA	Alveolar volume		
V̇A	Alveolar ventilation		
		WBC	White blood count
		WOB	Work of breathing

Metric Measurements

Linear		Weight		Volume	
kilometer (km)	m × 10³	kilogram (kg)	g × 10³	kiloliter	1 × 10³
decameter	m × 10	decagram	g × 10	decaliter	1 × 10
meter (m)		gram (g)		liter (L)	
decimeter	m × 10⁻¹	decigram	g × 10⁻¹	deciliter (dL)	1 × 10⁻¹
centimeter (cm)	m × 10⁻²	centigram	g × 10⁻²	centiliter	1 × 10⁻²
millimeter (mm)	m × 10⁻³	milligram (mg)	g × 10⁻³	milliliter (mL)	1 × 10⁻³
micrometer (μ or μm)	m × 10⁻⁶	microgram (μg)	g × 10⁻⁶	microliter (μL)	1 × 10⁻⁶

U.S. Customary and Metric Equivalents

1 inch	2.54 cm	1 ounce (oz)	28.35g	1 ounce (fl)	29.57 mL
1 foot	.0348 m	1 pound	454 g	1 quart	0.9463 L
1 mile	1.609 km	1 gram	0.0352 oz	1 gallon	3.785 L
1 micron	3.937 × 10⁻⁵ in	1 kilogram	2.2 lb	cubic inch	16.39 mL
1 centimeter	0.3937 in			cubic foot	28.32 L
1 meter	39.37 in			1 liter	1.057 qt
1 kilometer	0.6214 mile				61.02 in³
					0.03532 ft³

Conversion Tables

Temperature

°C = (°F-32) x 5/9   °F = (°C x 9/5) + 32

°F	°C	°C	°F
0	-17.7	0	32
95	35.0	35.0	95.0
96	35.5	35.5	95.9
97	36.1	36.0	96.8
98	36.6	36.5	97.7
99	37.2	37.0	98.6
100	37.7	37.5	99.5
101	38.3	38.0	100.4
102	38.8	38.5	101.3
103	39.4	39.0	102.2
104	40.0	39.5	103.1
105	40.5	40.0	104.0
106	41.1	40.5	104.9
107	41.6	41.0	105.8
108	42.2	41.5	106.6
109	42.7	42.0	107.6
110	43.3	100.0	212.0

Length

1 inch = 2.54 cm

inch	cm
1	2.5
2	5.1
4	10.2
6	15.2
8	20.3
12	30.5
18	46
24	61
30	76
36	91
42	107
48	122
54	137
60	152
66	168
72	183
78	198

Weight

1 lb = 0.454 kg   1 kg = 2.2 lb

lb	kg	kg	lb
1	0.5	1	2.2
2	0.9	2	4.4
4	1.8	3	6.6
6	2.7	4	8.8
8	3.6	5	11.0
10	4.5	6	13.2
20	9.1	8	17.6
30	13.6	10	22
40	18.3	20	44
50	22.7	30	66
60	27.3	40	88
70	31.8	50	110
80	36.4	60	132
90	40.9	70	154
100	45.4	80	176
150	69.2	90	198
200	90.8	100	220

Pressure

1.36cmH20 = 1 mmHg
1 cmH20 = 0.098 kPa
1 cmH20 = 0.735 kPa
1 mmHg = 0.133 kPa

cmH20	mmHg
6.8	5
13.6	10
20.4	15
27.2	20
33.9	25
40.7	30
47.5	35
54.3	40
61.1	45

1 PSIG	70.31 cmH20
1	760 mmHg
atmosphere	14.7 psi
	0 psi (gauge)
	1034 cmH20

Infection Control Guidelines

CDC Standard Precautions	
Applies to:	1) All patients (regardless of diagnosis or infection status).
	2) Blood, all body fluids, secretions, excretions (except sweat), non-intact skin, and mucous membranes.
Handwashing	Wash hands after; touching blood, body fluids, secretions, excretions, or contaminated items (even if wearing gloves); immediately after removing gloves; between patient contacts; between tasks/procedures on different body sites of the same patient; and when otherwise indicated. Use plain soap for routine handwashing and antimicrobial soap or waterless antiseptic for specific instances.
Gloves	Wear clean gloves when touching blood, body fluids, secretions, excretions, contaminated items, mucous membranes, and nonintact skin. Change gloves between tasks/procedures on same patient after contact within the infectious material. Remove gloves promptly after use, before touching noncontaminated items or surfaces, and before going to another patient. Wash hands immediately after removing gloves.
Gowns	Wear a clean gown to protect skin and clothing from splashes or sprays of blood, body fluids, secretions, or excretions. Remove soiled gown as promptly as possible and wash hands.
Patient Care Equipment	Handle used equipment soiled with blood, body fluids, secretions, and excretions in a manner that prevents skin and mucous membrane exposure, contamination of clothing, and transfer of microorganisms to other patients and/or environments. Do not use reusable equipment for another patient unless cleaned/reprocessed appropriately. Properly discard single-use items.
Occupational Health and Blood-borne Pathogens	Use extreme caution when handling, cleaning, or disposing of needles, scalpels, and other sharp instruments or devices. Never recap, use both hands, or point towards the body any used needles; rather, use either a one-handed "scoop" technique or a mechanical device. Do not bend, break, manipulate, or remove used needles from disposable syringes by hand. Place used disposable syringes and needles, scalpel blades, and other sharp items in appropriate puncture-resistant containers; place reusable syringes and needles in a puncture-resistant container for to be reprocessed. Use mouthpieces, resuscitation bags, or other ventilation devices as an alternative to mouth to mouth resuscitation.
Patient Placement	Use a private room for patients who contaminate the environment or who do not/cannot assist in maintaining appropriate hygiene or environmental control. Consult with infection control if a private room is not available.
Mask, Eye Protection, Face Shield:	Wear to protect eyes, nose, and mouth from splashes/sprays of blood/body fluids,/secretions/excretions.

Transmission-Based Precautions

Additional precautions beyond Standard Precautions.

Applies to: Patients with known or suspected infections (or colonized) with pathogens that can be transmitted by airborne, droplet, or contact.

Airborne Precautions (Small particle airborne droplet nuclei)	**Patient Placement:** Private negative-pressure room with 6 to12 air changes/hr, plus either safe external air discharge or HEPA filtration. Cohorting acceptable or consult with infection control. Keep room door closed and patient in room. **Patient Transport:** Essential purposes only. Have patient wear a surgical mask. **Respiratory Protection:** Wear N95 respirator when entering room of patient with known/suspected infectious pulmonary TB. Persons immune to measles (rubeola) or varicella (chickenpox) need not wear respiratory protection. If possible, persons not immune to measles or varicella should not enter the room, or wear respiratory protection.
Droplet Precautions (Large droplets)	**Patient Placement:** Private room, cohorting acceptable, or separate patient from others (patients and visitors) by > 3 feet. **Patient Transport:** Essential purposes only. Have patient wear a surgical mask. **Mask:** Wear a surgical mask within 3 ft. of patient (or upon entering room).
Contact Precautions (Hand or skin-to-skin contact)	**Patient Placement:** Private room, cohorting acceptable, or consult with infection control. **Patient Transport:** Essential purposes only. If must be transported, minimize risk of disease transmission. **Gloves and Handwashing:** Wear clean gloves upon entering room. Change gloves after contact with infectious material. Remove gloves before leaving patient's environment and wash hands immediately with antimicrobial agent or waterless antiseptic. Then do not touch any potentially contaminated surface or item. **Gown:** Wear clean gown upon entering room if anticipate patient, surface, or item contact; if patient incontinent, has diarrhea, ileostomy, colostomy, or wound drainage not contained by a dressing. Remove gown before leaving room, then do not contact any potentially contaminated surface. **Patient Care Equipment:** Dedicate use of noncritical equipment to single patient or cohort. If shared, ensure adequately cleaned and disinfected before next patient use.

* Guideline for Isolation Precautions: Preventing Transmission of Infectious Agents in Healthcare Settings 2007. http://www.cdc.gov/ncidod/dhqp/pdf/guidelines/Isolation2007.pdf

Index

Xolair 12-27
Xopenex 12-17

Z

zafirlukast 12-15
zanamivir 12-25
Zemaira 12-22
zileuton 12-15
Zyban 12-32
Zyflo 12-15

Notes:

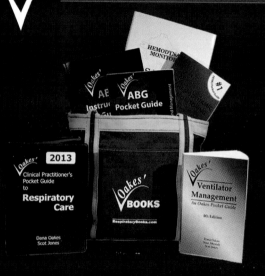